HEALTH CARE
MELTDOWN

Dr. E. Smith's
PATENT
MAGNETIC
INDUCTOR.

If not called for in 10 days P. M. return to
Dr. E. SMITH, Normal, Ills.

HEALTH CARE MELTDOWN

CONFRONTING THE MYTHS AND FIXING OUR FAILING SYSTEM

Robert H. LeBow, M.D.

Foreword by
John P. Geyman, M.D.
Afterword by
Don McCanne, M.D.

Alan C. Hood & Company, Inc.
CHAMBERSBURG, PENNSYLVANIA
2004

The patent medicine illustrations in the book were printed on mailing envelopes, a popular advertising device in the 19th century. The original envelopes are a part of the postal history collection of Bob LeBow.

The cures were peddled to the public by a group sometimes referred to as *snake oil merchants*, who created a mythology of misinformation in order to enhance their own economic interests.

Manufactured in the United States of America

Published by Alan C. Hood & Co., Inc.
P. O. Box 775, Chambersburg, PA 17201

Library of Congress cataloging-in-publication data
LeBow, Robert H., 1940-
    Health care meltdown : confronting the myths & fixing our failing system / Robert H. LeBow ; foreword by John P. Geyman.
        p. cm.
    Includes bibliographical references and index.
    ISBN 0-911469-23-0 (paperback)
    1. Medical care—United States—Evaluation. 2. Medical policy—United States—Evaluation. 3. Social medicine—United States. 4. Medicine—United States. I. Title.

RA395.A3L413 2003
362.1'0973—dc21

                                                                                            2003049911

ISBN 0-911469-23-0

10 9 8 7 6 5 4 3 2 1

Dedicated to the memory of
TERRY REILLY,
my partner in the struggle for
Health Care for All

Contents

Part I: The Problem
A Wasteful, Dysfunctional System and a Nation Kept Clueless

Part II: Towards Finding a Solution

Foreword

IT IS NOW WIDELY RECOGNIZED that the U.S. health care "system" is seriously ill. With 43 million uninsured and many millions of Americans underinsured or insecurely insured, escalating health care costs are pricing health care services beyond the reach of a large and growing part of the population. Although the U.S. spends far more on health care than any other country in the world, our health care is of inconsistent quality, many countries have better outcomes of care, and the system is stifled by bureaucracy and administrative complexity.

Admittedly, the health care system is extremely complex, but a major driver of uncontrollable health care inflation is the market-based system itself. Although it has been well known for many years that health care markets do not behave like other markets in the economy in controlling costs through competition, the nation continues on its market-based approach, now largely controlled by a small number of large health care corporations. Medicine and health care have been transformed by corporate interests with an overriding mission of maximizing profits for themselves and their shareholders. The long tradition of public service in health care has been compromised.

Although incremental attempts to reform the system have failed for over 30 years, we continue to be assured by legislators, politicians and health policy "experts" that one or another new incremental change to the market-based system will improve access and control costs. This message is amplified through the media and lobbyist efforts of corporate stakeholders in the status quo. The prevailing political view today touts the promise of a consumer choice model, but this translates to shifting the increasingly unaffordable costs of health care from employers, insurers, and even the government, to consumers themselves. The present system is not sustainable without fundamental reform.

Health insurance coverage is the single most important requirement to assure access to health care. All other industrialized Western nations adopted one or another form of social health insurance long ago.

In the U.S., however, an enormous, largely for-profit insurance industry "cherry picks" the market, favoring the healthy and avoiding the sick through outright denials or risk-based premium increases. The insurance industry and other investor-owned health care corporations join forces in blocking any reforms that would regulate their prices or threaten their prerogatives.

Health care reform is again a central issue on the domestic agenda as the 2004 election campaigns heat up. The publication of Dr. Bob LeBow's book, *Health Care Meltdown*, could not be more timely. He has dedicated his career to community-based primary care and social justice in health care. In this book, he combines this experience with many years of study of the health care system. He has given us a real-world portrait of the problems and inequities of today's system, presented in such an insightful and readable way that the inescapable lessons shine through.

It is ironic and tragic that Dr. LeBow, a lifelong athlete and dedicated cyclist, was rendered quadriplegic after a bicycle accident in 2002, even though he was wearing a helmet. He never lost his passion for health care reform. He spoke at an August 2003 news conference in Philadelphia as a strong advocate of a notional health insurance program. His untimely death three months later at age 63 was a great loss to the country's growing movement toward social justice in health care, but his words live on in his writings—"It is time to put the patient first—not last—in the setting of priorities."

It has been said that we are entitled to our own interpretations, but not to our own facts. Here, in Dr. LeBow's well-researched book, we have undeniable facts which point to needed reforms. His book is a testimonial to the failure of incremental change, and we are given a realistic and compelling prescription for change. This book will be of great interest to everyone involved in planning, delivery or evaluation of health care, as well as policy makers, legislators, and lay readers concerned about our failing health care system and the urgent need for reform.

John P. Geyman, M.D.
Professor Emeritus of Family Medicine
University of Washington Medical School
Seattle, Washington
February 2004

Prologue

THIRTY YEARS AGO, AS I was heading toward a career in international health, I became aware of how poorly our American health care system was working. I saw how millions of our own people were being denied the care they needed. And I began to appreciate how those same people were being robbed of their dignity.

In 1971 I had completed a two-year stint as a Peace Corps physician in Bolivia, and the following year I finished a Master's in Public Health course in international health at Johns Hopkins. It was then that I decided to switch my geographic focus and work with our own "third world" right here in America.

I moved my family to Idaho to join a migrant health center that had just received its initial grant, and I became its first medical director. In an old grocery store that had been purchased for $6000, and in a variety of makeshift venues like church basements, I helped organize and run a series of health centers that served poor people, then largely migrant farmworkers, in southwest Idaho. Mostly I took care of patients. As a family practitioner, I did everything from obstetrics to geriatrics. Over 30 years I delivered almost 2000 babies. I've followed some of the same patients for three decades, long enough to deliver babies for women I'd help to bring into the world 20 years earlier. And I've helped to train scores of health care professionals including nurse practitioners, physician assistants, medical students, and residents.

In the mid-'80s I began to wonder about what I was doing. Despite all the sleep deprivation I could handle, my patients and I were still hitting the same stone wall when it came to dealing with our health care system. Despite all our efforts as a "safety-net" community health center, people were still forced to go without needed care. They were still being robbed of their dignity. I was still having to "beg, borrow, and steal" to get care for my patients. And I came to the realization that change was not going to come unless our nation changed how it looked at health care and at ourselves as a nation. Americans were not going to regain their dignity unless our nation changed.

It was a personal tragedy that inspired me, directly and indirectly, to become a health care activist. In 1986 my younger son Tommy died at age 16 in an auto accident. He might have survived if he had been wearing his seat belt. Without exaggerating, I calculated that I had told him to put his seat belt on at least 2000 times. A month after his death, the Idaho State Legislature was holding hearings on a new seat belt law for Idaho. I testified before committees in both the House and the Senate. The law would not have passed had I not spoken up. It passed the House by only three votes, and I received letters from three representatives who said they changed their vote because of my testimony.

As a result of my son's untimely death, through a series of unusual circumstances, I also became a columnist for our local newspaper, now *The Idaho Press-Tribune*. I kept that job for eight years, and I wrote a column every week—any subject I wanted, at six dollars a column—except when I was campaigning for political office.

More poignantly, with Tommy's death there was also a more personal feeling that motivated me to become an activist. I felt responsible to do whatever I could to help others avoid the kind of sorrow and grief that comes with, for example, the death of a child.

Inspired to enter politics to change the raw deal my patients were getting with their health care, I ran for a House seat in the Idaho State Legislature—three times. I picked the wrong party to win, but I learned a lot about politics. In one election campaign, I knocked on the doors of close to 3000 households. And I got to listen to the gripes of a lot of people. In 1988, I became active with Physicians for a National Health Program (PNHP), a national organization striving for universal coverage through national health insurance. For two years, in 1998 and 1999, I was president of that organization.

While I continue to work at my community health center in Idaho, since January 2001 I've become a half-time "health care activist." Like many of my fellow activists, I spend long hours preparing and making presentations to a variety of groups, planning initiatives, organizing and attending meetings, writing articles, and generally trying to drum up support for universal coverage for health care. In my quest, I've found that one of the greatest obstacles to meaningful health care reform is the degree to which we Americans are clueless about our health care system. Most Americans—including politicians and even knowledgeable health care professionals who should know better—have been led down an assortment of primrose paths. They have been sucked into arguing about the fine points of a variety of diversions such as the nearly irrelevant "patient protection" debate. They have even been led to give serious consideration to options that would make our disaster of a health system even more complex and unresponsive.

I see my patients continuing to wander in the health care wilderness, without much hope of finding the path out. Even more ominous, I see millions of currently insured Americans facing the danger of losing their coverage—and their dignity—as our health care system slips towards "meltdown." The options I see being proposed offer a few crumbs to my patients and increasing obstacles for everyone else, but no lasting solution. And I see these options being justified by the usual host of myths that have been used for decades to derail meaningful health care reform.

Until we can confront the myths and choose a real solution that provides affordable, comprehensive health care for every person in America, an ever-increasing number of middle-class Americans will join my low-income patients in health care limbo. Middle-class folks' misadventures with health care will increasingly resemble the stories of the uninsured and underinsured that I have related in this book. Middle-class Americans are already quietly acquiescing to a growing number of indignities foisted upon them by our failing system. And they are learning to accept the type of rationing endured by my uninsured patients: health care that is delayed or skipped altogether. As we approach another crossroads for our American health care system, I fear that more and more Americans will suffer unnecessary pain and illness, as well as increasing humiliation.

I am passionate on the issues because my passion is rekindled on a daily basis as I struggle with my patients to jump through unnecessary and wasteful hoops to meet their health care needs. I have tried to remain objective in what I describe. However, I have deliberately strayed from an academic approach because, in dealing with the problems involved in health care reform, I am trying to concentrate more on some of the deeper and more human dimensions that are not addressed in the usual academic or economic studies.

I have drawn many examples from my Idaho experience, where I have been practicing for many years. If anything, the situation for health care is worse elsewhere, especially in large urban areas where the indignities can be perpetrated with more anonymity. Idaho remains a small state where personal connections still count, and Idaho has had the good fortune of being largely passed over by the "managed-care revolution." But even in Idaho, I'm seeing the increasing burden being laid upon middle-class people, people with insurance, insurance that is becoming progressively more inadequate.

This book is an attempt to bring to light some of the myths that are obstructing change and to propose a solution so that every person in America (including my patients) can get the health care he or she needs. In this richest of all countries, we have the resources, both economic and human, to change the quagmire that our health care system has become. What we lack is the vision, the political will, and the courage to stand up to the vested interests.

Bob LeBow, M.D., MPH
Boise, Idaho
July 2002

Acknowledgements

I want to thank profusely those people who laboriously plowed through early draft versions of this book. Without their help, this work would not have been possible. Their advice and direction have been invaluable. I am especially grateful to Marcia Bondy, Ed Crawford, Maria Eschen, Ellen Kurnit, David Reese, Julia Robinson, and Todd Swanson for their perseverance in giving me enlightened feedback. To my brother, Joel LeBow, I owe a special thanks, for reading the whole draft document at a single sitting, and then getting back to me with insightful comments from a consumer's point of view.

I also owe special thanks to my wife of 40 years, Gail, who has provided ongoing critical suggestions as well as unwavering support for this project. Thanks also go to my "technical support" team, including Jennifer LeBow, Nicole LeFavour, and Jean Miller.

With respect to the issue of health care in America, and my involvement in the "cause" of Health Care for All, I'd like to thank Don McCanne, for his informative e-mail network "Quote of the Day," which has provided many useful leads; Physicians for a National Health Program, which has supplied a host of useful data and information; the late Terry Reilly, who recruited me in 1972 to work with migrant farmworkers in Idaho; his wife Rosie Delgadillo Reilly, who, for more than 30 years, has been a champion of the underserved; colleagues in my practice, who have provided me with "stories of the uninsured and under-insured"; innumerable other colleagues, all involved in the "cause" as well, who have provided me with thought-provoking ideas and inspiration; and my patients, who have been gracious enough to share their experiences and ideas with me.

HEALTH CARE
MELTDOWN

Dr. E. Smith's PATENT MAGNETIC INDUCTOR

Dr. E. SMITH, Normal, Ills.

Confronting the Myths:
Can America Halt the Slide Toward
Health Care Meltdown?

Rigoberto sat nervously on the edge of the exam table and broke into tears. A large and reserved 17-year-old, he had asthma and a nasty cough that hadn't improved in two weeks. I was about to prescribe an inhaler and antibiotics. "What's wrong?" I asked. He glanced at his mother. "On our way here, I found out we didn't have money to pay for the visit," he said, wiping his eyes with the back of his hand.

I reassured him that, since we were a community health center, money wasn't a problem. I forewarned our pharmacy to give him the prescriptions without pressing for payment. But after I left the exam room, our collections person entered and politely asked for eight dollars, our "nominal" fee. Mother and son broke into tears of embarrassment and left without the medications.

AMERICAN HEALTH CARE IS once again at a "crossroads," one of several windows of opportunity for change that we have had over the past 90 years. The last "opportunity moment" in American health care—marked by President Clinton's ill-fated and ill-conceived "managed-competition" proposal—ended in 1994 with the collapse of his plan. Since then, we have had a vacuum in leadership and direction. "Market" principles and the pursuit of profit have become the norm for health care. Cost shifting from employers to employees has accelerated, and access to care has become more difficult. The number of uninsured Americans has grown and now, with the economic

1

downturn, is increasing even more. America's brief "managed-care revolution," with its temporary slowing of some health care costs, is dead. The American public would no longer put up with being exploited and abused by managed-care organizations. As for the uninsured, their situation has only become worse.

As we approach this new crossroads for health care, our system is failing and in imminent danger of collapse or "meltdown." Fortunately, for the moment, the system is still capable of meeting the health care needs of many who find themselves in a crisis. We have wonderful technology. There are thousands of dedicated and caring clinicians and others who try their best to help people in need. But more and more the needs of people are not being met. The number of Americans without adequate access to care is growing. More and more, Americans are delaying care or going without needed services. They show up at a crisis stage in increasingly beleaguered emergency rooms.

Hospitals are overcrowded and understaffed. Over 90 percent of our nursing homes have an inadequate number of nurses. Ambulances circle around waiting for an open spot at an emergency room. Medical errors happen much too frequently. Costs are soaring. Patient expectations are soaring too, as new technologies and drugs become available. Waste abounds as money that could be used for patient care is instead diverted to pay for higher administrative costs that are a result of the increasing (and unnecessary) complexity and "gaming" of our system. Our federal programs, Medicare and Medicaid, are endangered. There is no planning, no vision for the future, as our nonsystem seems to be imploding.

Millions of Americans, the 40+ million without health insurance, have been deprived of their dignity, and we're in danger of losing our dignity as a nation. America is the only developed nation that fails to guarantee access to needed care for all its citizens and the only advanced country that permits someone to go bankrupt because of poor health. Even Americans who have health insurance are increasingly being squeezed or sometimes forced to forego care, as depicted somewhat melodramatically in the recent movie "John Q." A survey done at the end of 2001 showed that 43 percent of Americans with private insurance feared that their family's insurance coverage might be eliminated or reduced in the next year.[1]

Millions of Americans have become "health care beggars."[2] Millions more, including middle-class Americans, are at risk of joining them as beggars in the near future as the cost of health care soars.

Our Poor Performance and Perverse Incentives

DESPITE OUR STANDING AS the richest country in the world—and despite our spending nearly twice as much per person on health care than any other country—the overall results have been disappointing, dehumanizing, and at times even abysmal. Our health status indicators rank us near the bottom among the developed countries in such measures as life expectancy and infant mortality. In 2000 the World Health Organization ranked the U.S. health care system at number 37 overall.

Meanwhile, our population grows more obese and sedentary. Substance abuse continues at a high rate. Failure to deal adequately with mental health has contributed to our burgeoning prison population. And debt from health care is now the second highest reason for personal bankruptcy. The pursuit of profit has assumed primacy over the pursuit of what is best for people.

Why the disconnect? Where have we failed? Does anybody care?

Our health care system—or, more precisely, nonsystem—has evolved into a monster, a disorganized, overly complex creature that robs people of their health, their money and their dignity. Yet the great majority of Americans are unaware—or clueless—of what has happened to America's health care. Blind belief in certain icons of American economic theory—icons that have limited relevance to health care—have helped cause our current dilemma.

Faith in "the market" and competition, stress on "personal responsibility" and individualism, and dislike of government regulation or managed anything have contributed to the creation of a system which turns a blind eye to millions of patients like

Rigoberto who "do without." We Americans live in a milieu of purposeful health care ignorance. Merchants of misinformation and myth spend millions of dollars to keep us clueless. By doing so, they limit improvements in our health care system to piecemeal bits of change. Remember Harry and Louise? The bus from Canada? Citizens for a Better Medicare? They're only a few of the scams perpetrated on the American public by the vested interests. By delaying or averting a comprehensive solution, the health care entrepreneurs prolong the time they are able to reap profits from the system. Profits they keep for themselves and their shareholders while my patients, and millions more like them, are forced to become "health care beggars" or "go without."

A large part of our problem stems from the perverse incentives of the system. For much too long, America's health care system has been driven (on the supply side) by self-interest. Instead of commitment to community and cooperation, the overriding ethic of health care in America has become self-interest and the pursuit of profit. The American people have been left out of the equation. Even worse, they have been systematically duped and then blamed for being "overutilizers" by some of the same special-interest groups that misled them. Americans are told to exercise more "personal responsibility," a code word for shifting costs to the consumer. But they have been set up by the health care industry (insurers, drug companies, medical establishment) to have high expectations and to create a demand for expensive goods and services. As for the people who can't afford the expensive services, they don't matter. There are no profits to be made from the poor, unless they can qualify for a government program that will pay their bills.

The Search for a Comprehensive Solution

AN INTEREST IN UNIVERSAL coverage once again seems to be growing, though it appears to be morphing into a less ambitious goal of "reducing the number" of the uninsured. Some of the factors creating pressure for health care reform include an economic recession, a growing unemployment rate, and the accelerating costs of health care. Health insurance premium rates rose by 11 percent in 2001 and are expected to rise 15 percent in 2002. The events of 9/11 also may have reawakened some sense of community in America as well as a questioning of the axiom that less government is always better. There is also a growing sense of despair from the ever-increasing number of Americans who are hurting from being *under*insured. Including the 40 million uninsured Americans, we are reaching perhaps a critical mass of people, a total of maybe as many as 90 million (not even including Medicare beneficiaries), who need help. With the growing number of people in distress, including many more middle-class Americans, there is bound to be a more strident demand for change.

Groups (such as the insurance industry, the pharmaceutical companies, and some elements of the medical care establishment) with special financial interests in our health care system will likely continue to play games of disinformation to derail significant change. And they will twist the mantra of "personal responsibility" to make people believe that financial barriers to care, like increased deductibles and co-pays, are good for them. They will invoke the "mantra" of "socialized medicine" to attack any increased role for government. Yet government needs to have a role—at the very least in oversight, coordination, and leadership—if we are to fix our failing health care system.

We are hearing increasingly about incremental or "piece-meal" reforms, about vouchers, tax credits, medical savings accounts, and "defined contributions" from employers. There are now a plethora of ideas about how to "cover more Americans." Most of them are complex, and some experts argue that we may have to make our system more complex than it already is. But people who have been working within the system, and who appreciate the abuses and loss of dignity suffered by so many Americans seeking adequate health care, know these "piece-meal" solutions will only prolong the agony and maintain the status quo. And the status quo has become increasingly intolerable as our system heads toward meltdown.

Getting America Clued In

I'VE WRITTEN THIS BOOK in an effort to shed light on the degree of cluelessness that permeates American health care. I have attempted to use my 30 years of experience working within a dysfunctional health system and my efforts as a health care activist to sort out the realities and the myths. I am concerned that the "piecemeal" direction in which we seem to be headed will not help *my* patients or the millions of other Americans who are likely to join their ranks as "health care beggars." I worry that even friendly allies who advocate for "doing something" will compromise the chances for millions of Americans to get the health care they need. If even a few million Americans are left hanging in limbo, our nation will not have regained its dignity.

I have not included lengthy economic analyses. Instead, I have provided a selective bibliography that readers can refer to for more detailed information. I have tried to concentrate on an analysis of the key issues that we must address to achieve meaningful reform. I have also attempted to provide an *ad hoc* type of road map for reaching the goal. Some of the principal themes that I address in this book include:

- The high degree of misinformation and myth that has been intentionally used by what I have termed the "modern-day snake oil merchants" to hawk their products and discredit system changes that might limit their influence or profits.

- The twisted "market" model as it has been applied to health care. How, instead of putting the customer first, it has in fact put the patient last.

- How the "personal responsibility" mantra and co-pays/deductibles act as barriers to care and are used to "blame the victims" and shift cost or increase profits.

- How we need to think more in terms of societal or community responsibility.

- A smattering of real patient experiences: misadventures

of the uninsured and the underinsured. (All the names have been changed.)

- How Americans have missed the boat on prevention and what we must do about it.

- Affordability, and the poor value we get for our health care investment in America, especially compared to other developed nations.

- What direction do we need to take at this crossroads? How can we arrive at a solution that is really universal and affordable and provides *everyone* with the health care they need?

- The importance of "one risk pool"—and not lip service to "pluralism"—in reaching a universal coverage that is fair and affordable and does not exclude the sick.

- Some humility in admitting that health care alone cannot give America good health, that it takes a wider approach involving social and economic change, including efforts at prevention, to reach good health.

- That Health Care for All is a key first step in returning dignity to individuals, families, and our nation, and that, without it, we will be unable to resolve the gaping health disparities that we have in America today.

"One Risk Pool"/ National Health Insurance

I BELIEVE THAT UNLESS America chooses a solution that incorporates the concept of "one risk pool," such as national health insurance, we will never solve our dilemma. Former Senator Bob Kerry expressed his support for this approach when he testified before the Senate Finance Committee in March 2002.[3] He advised against adding a prescription drug benefit to Medicare— "not unless you are prepared to make fundamental changes in the way Americans finance the cost of their health care." He went on to assert:

"Beginning with a universal entitlement does not mean higher spending or more governmental interference with the choices made by patients or providers. In truth, it could mean a lot less of both. It would mean that we would start thinking about ourselves as a single group of 280 million Americans who are all part of the same health system and who all need to face the challenge of matching our appetite for quality with our capacity to pay."

Perhaps there are solutions other than national health insurance—or its equivalent—for America to achieve universal coverage in a way that is both comprehensive and affordable. It's possible that we could model a solution after approaches adopted by some European countries and express the goal as "assuring universal access to care for all needed medical services." However, as described in the chapters that follow, it is difficult to imagine how there could be a fairer, more efficient approach than "one risk pool" that would truly cover *every* person in America. The type of solution envisaged in this book is embodied in this concept. "One risk pool" is virtually synonymous with what is referred to as a "single-payer" approach, though they are not precisely the same since "one risk pool" refers more to the group of people covered as opposed to a payment mechanism.

Under "one risk pool" (see the Appendix for a brief summary of "frequently asked questions" about "one risk pool") everybody in America would be covered in the same health insurance plan. There would be no questions about enrollment or eligibility. Since the largest possible number of people would be "pooled together," there would be economies of scale. There would be no more "cherry-picking," no more excluding of the poor or the sick from access to needed care. No one would go bankrupt because of medical bills. Savings from the elimination of middlemen and other administrative costs would allow every person coverage with a comprehensive package of benefits without increasing our overall spending on health care.

Instead of premiums, co-pays, and deductibles, the plan would be funded through progressive taxation and would have a trust fund specifically devoted to the plan, much like today's Medicare. There would be a larger government role in collecting the taxes and overseeing the plan. But the delivery system would remain predominantly private, as it is today. Each person would be able to choose any provider of services he or she chose, in effect *increasing* choice. "One risk pool" refers to the financing mechanism only, has no direct effect on the delivery system, and does not in any way diminish the role of the private sector in providing health care. It is not socialized medicine. It is a way to minimize administrative costs and create equity.

The general principles that comprise this approach, which would in effect be a form of national health insurance, include the following:

- *True universality. Everybody in, nobody out, with one risk pool. No more "cherry-picking," or exclusion of high-risk people from coverage.*

- *Tax-based financing, like Medicare, in accordance with income, instead of premiums, deductibles, and co-pays. Not free care, since everybody pays into the system through taxes.*

- *Full choice of providers in a delivery system that remains a mix of private and public. Not socialized medicine, but national health insurance in the same way Medicare is a national insurance program.*

- *Elimination of the odd link between employers and health insurance coverage.*

- *Coverage for all necessary services, including inpatient and outpatient care, emergency care, long-term care, mental health, treatment for substance abuse, prescriptions, and basic dental and eye care with no discrimination by type of illness or ability to pay.*

- *True integration of public health and preventive services with adequate funding, both on a personal and community basis.*

- *Continued funding for the special services necessary to serve special population groups; e.g., immigrants, migrant farm workers, and the disabled.*

- *The practice of medicine based on scientific principles.*

- *A national trust fund dedicated specifically to health care.*

- *National planning that allows a high degree of local autonomy. A national health board with regional or state-by-state equivalents.*

- *Public accountability. Eliminates the "opaque"(hard to fathom) financing practices of the current system.*

- *Global budgeting, which entails setting priorities, but is flexible enough to support medical education, research, and excellence in medicine.*

- *Simplified administration with greatly reduced administrative costs, leaving 90–95 percent of health care funds for patient care, prevention, and research.*

- *Reasonable and equitable reimbursement for health care providers.*

- *Insurance companies would be allowed to sell policies only for uncovered services.*

- *Treatment of health as a "public good" instead of as a market commodity.*

PART ONE

The Problem

A Wasteful,
Dysfunctional System,
and a Nation Kept
Clueless

Chapter 1

Myths, Misinformation, and the Pursuit of Profit

America has the best health care system in the world.
— Many American politicians

The moon is made of green cheese.
— Anonymous, 16th Century, likely a dairyman

IN THE ANTHOLOGY OF myths about health care in America, there is the "Alpha Myth" that asserts "America has the best health care system in the world." It is heard over and over, most frequently from the mouths of politicians. Many Americans, not knowing any better, believe it. This and a host of other myths about health care in America have arisen partly out of ignorance and partly from our insularity.

There is a national sentiment that (of course) America must be the best in almost everything. So it is with health care. Playing on Americans' assumption of superiority, special interests with major financial stakes in our health care sector have made certain to reinforce and spread the mantra that we have "the best health care system in the world." The more the American people can be lulled into accepting this mantra, the more the special interests can continue to exploit the system to their own advantage and profit.

Facts belie these myths, however. As Stephen Bezruchka,[1] Barbara Starfield [2] and others have pointed out, the United States does very poorly when it comes to the standard measurements of health status. In fact, we rank about 20th or lower when com-

13

pared with other developed nations in such measures as life expectancy, infant mortality, and immunizations.

Much of this disparity comes from the ever-widening gap in America between the rich and the poor. Bezruchka even theorizes that the wide gap itself is the reason for the differences. America has a higher percentage of people living in poverty than most other developed countries. And America, unlike all the other developed countries, has not embraced the principle that health care should be a basic human right. In America, health care is a privilege, not a right.

The 2000 World Health Organization (WHO) report on the world's health care systems[3] ranked the U.S. 37th "overall." We scored low in other categories as well, such as in "fairness," where the U.S. ranked 54th, tied with Fiji. However, we came in first (by far) in "spending." Very likely we also have the world's best technology, which Americans can access if they're able to pay for it. And we also are unique in having a fragmented, inefficient, and administratively wasteful system that excludes one-seventh of our population from insurance coverage.

A Myriad of Myths

BESIDES THE FALSE MANTRA that "America has the best health care system in the world," there are many other oft-cited myths about health care in America. These are used to promote a variety of political or economic agendas. They include but are not limited to:

1) We don't have a problem with access to care in America since anyone can get needed health care by going to an emergency room.

2) The system's not broken, so it doesn't need to be fixed.

3) "The market" can solve the problems with our health care system.

4) Private solutions are always better than public solutions.

5) Medicare is going broke.

6) America can't afford universal coverage.

7) Americans will not accept health care "rationing" like they have in other countries.

8) Canada's health care system is terrible and failing.

9) The insured are subsidizing the care of the uninsured.

10) We don't have the resources to handle the increased demand for services that would result from universal coverage.

11) Drug prices are higher in the U.S. because our pharmaceutical industry spends billions of dollars on research and development.

12) We can get to universal coverage through incremental or piecemeal change.

13) Americans will never accept a "single-payer" system.

Myth #1: Everybody Has Access to Care Through the Emergency Room

WE DON'T HAVE A problem with access to care in America since anyone can get needed health care by going to an emergency room. Unfortunately, way too many Americans are forced to use emergency rooms (ERs) to obtain their health care. Many people, especially the uninsured, lack a regular health care provider and have nowhere else to go. But the ERs are the most expensive and inefficient way to deliver primary care.

For example, consider a person with a urinary tract infection or bronchitis. Going to the ER instead of a primary care provider often ends up with a two- to four-hour wait and a bill for $500. If that person had gone to a primary care clinician, it probably would have been an hour wait and a bill closer to $80. Moreover, the ER physician usually does not know the patient, has no previous medical records, and is much more obliged to practice defensive medicine (i.e., more expensive, with more tests). Follow up is incomplete and uncertain. The patient is often given a few sample pills and a prescription to take to a pharmacy only to find they can't afford to buy the medicine.

Emergency rooms are being stressed to the maximum. *U.S.A. Today* published a front-page story[4] about how the ERs in the U.S. were falling apart under the strain of too many patients. This scenario now plays out each winter (the season for high patient demand) at many ERs in cities throughout America.

ERs are being inappropriately used for primary care in America because our system to deliver primary care is inadequate. Only in recent years has there been an increase in outpatient "urgent care" or "doc-in-the-box" clinics offering extended hours of service. But these clinics lack continuity of care. They deal only with the immediate problem.

We saw a young uninsured woman who had gone to one of these clinics for a severe kidney infection. She was treated appropriately, given a shot of an antibiotic and a prescription for Cipro. She bought the Cipro for $129, but two days later was still not feeling better. It turned out that her infection was resistant to Cipro but sensitive to Septra, an $8 medicine. She was concerned that she wouldn't be able to afford the cheaper medicine because she only had $2 left after paying for the Cipro. Fortunately we were able to give her what she needed.

A particularly disingenuous myth related to the "access to care through the ER" myth is that, since anyone can get care through an ER, the uninsured in America are in fact not suffering adverse effects to their health. The data to the contrary are overwhelming. They are summarized in a report released in 2000 by the American College of Physicians-American Society of Internal Medicine: "No Health Insurance? It's Enough to Make You Sick—Scientific Research Linking the Lack of Health Coverage to Poor Health."[5]

The Kaiser Commission on Medicaid and the Uninsured came out with a similar report in May 2002. Entitled "Sicker and Poorer: The Consequences of Being Uninsured," their report documents how being uninsured *does* matter. Through an extensive literature search, they show (among other findings) that the uninsured (1) have a 10 to 15 percent higher mortality rate and (2) earn 10 to 30 percent less because of their poor health.[6] Also in May 2002, the Institute of Medicine released the second of a series of six reports on the consequences of uninsurance. Entitled

Care Without Coverage: Too Little, Too Late, the study estimates that over 18,000 adults die each year in the U.S. because of the lack of health insurance.[7]

Myth #2: We Don't Need to Fix What's Not Broken

THE SYSTEM'S NOT BROKEN, so it doesn't need to be fixed. A favorite theme of some right-wing pundits is to deny that America has a health care crisis. This line of rhetoric assumes that the system must be functioning well since it works for 85 or 90 percent of Americans. It is still true that, for people with good health insurance and good connections to our health care system, the quality of the care they receive can be excellent. In an opinion piece that appeared in *American Medical News,* Richard F. Corlin, MD, the president of the AMA, extolled the medical care he received when he was traveling and suffered a collapsed lung. He concluded that, "...Most of our health delivery system is working very well and should not be discarded under the guise of correcting the problems of the uninsured or any other aspects of health care that need our attention."[8]

He's partially correct—and lucky. Many of our caregivers are competent and dedicated. But we have major problems with medical errors, poor access to care, the failure to practice scientific-based medicine, and the lack of a preventive approach to health care. However, it's primarily the financing system, and every aspect that relates to that system, that's failing. And the financing of health care drives the delivery system. In any given year, the great majority of Americans experience only minimal interface with our system. For example, the healthiest 20 percent of Americans spend only about $14 a year on health care. They have little to complain about, so they can be included in the "satisfied" category. But there are many millions of Americans who are not so healthy and, unlike Dr. Corlin, do not have good insurance or the savvy to work a system that can be very complex and frustrating.

We're failing the most with the uninsured, the 15 percent of Americans for whom the system does *not* work. Add to that number the additional 50 million or so Americans who are *under-insured*. These two groups of people often are the ones who need the care the most. They include many people with chronic diseases and "preexisting conditions" who are unable to afford insurance. Many of the uninsured don't even bother to show up for care unless they're critically ill. They are the "invisible uninsured."[9][10] Can our society really accept a "margin of error" of 15 percent or more when the result is serious disability or death? That's what we're doing today with health care. We're playing Russian roulette with the lives of the uninsured and, increasingly, the *under*insured.

Myth #3: "The Market" Is the Solution

"THE MARKET" CAN SOLVE the problems with our health care system. Americans are led to believe that faith in "the market" is the American way and that, given a chance, "the market" can solve anything. However, since the demise of the Clinton Plan in 1994 and the leadership vacuum that followed, we've had a chance to see what the market could do for health care.

With respect to the financing of health care, "the market" has been an abject failure. The market may work well with automobiles, housing, and fast food. But buying health care is a far cry from buying a hamburger. The much-vaunted advantage of market "competition" in health care has only resulted in increased woes for providers and patients. With competition being almost exclusively based on cost, the result has been the creation of oligopolies, the control of the market by large corporations.

Although managed care did lead to a temporary flattening of health care cost inflation, the effect was short-lived. It was mostly due to cutting back on provider reimbursements and denying care to patients. Managed-care organizations underpriced their products to gain market share and, as a result, half of them lost money in the late '90s. Many continue to lose money today. Moreover, the popular backlash to the abuses of managed care forced managed-care organizations to abandon many of their rationing mechanisms. Maybe the forces of competition could lead to better outcomes if quality were the issue, but with cost and profits as the motivators, "the market" in health care has led to:

- An increase in the uninsured. The number of uninsured went from 37 million to 43 million. Though there was a temporary drop in 1999-2000 (mostly due to the low rate of unemployment), the number is again rising rapidly. With the 2001 recession and the events of 9/11, Families USA estimated that in 2001 2.2 million Americans lost health care coverage due to increased unemployment alone.

- Despite rhetoric to the contrary, we saw a marked decrease in choice, as opposed to other developed countries where choice has been increasing.

- Markedly increased diversion of resources to administration, marketing, and profits, with less money left for patient care. Overall administrative costs in the U.S. are now estimated at 25 to 50 percent, with the highest rates being in areas where the "penetration" of managed care is the highest.

- A decrease in the quality of care and an increase in medical errors as cost saving became the main priority.

- A failure to deal with some of the more pressing—but less profitable—aspects of health care, such as mental health and public health. The failure to fund public health adequately became particularly evident when our nation was recently faced with the anthrax scare. This aspect of the failure of "the market" is extensively discussed in a book by Laurie Garrett.[11]

- An expansion of for-profit HMOs, a phenomenon that has come to be almost as reviled as the tobacco industry in America.

- Millions of dissatisfied Americans.

- Frustrated physicians because administrative demands have limited the amount of time they are able to spend with patients.

Myth #4: Private Is Always Better Than Public

PRIVATE SOLUTIONS ARE ALWAYS *better than public solutions.* Discrediting government has become (for some, at least) a popular American sport, along with (for some health care providers) ripping off government health care programs. Keeping the anti-government myth alive (e.g., "You don't want the government in your medicine cabinet, do you?") is an important element in maintaining control for a private sector that has excelled at manipulating regulations to maximize profits, as the pharmaceutical and energy (e.g., Enron) industries have done.

There is a subgroup of physicians—some would have us believe they are more numerous than they actually are—who are fiercely anti-government. In its July 2001 issue, the editor of *Physician's Money Digest* summed up their position on health care. He asserted that, "Most sensible physicians believe the key to correcting our health care trouble is to empower patients and physicians and to remove government interference." The patient counterpart for these "sensible" physicians might be the famous Florida senior who, during the campaign debates about the future of Medicare, angrily declared, "I don't want the government messing with my Medicare!" There is a love-hate relationship here. Seniors overwhelmingly support Medicare, yet there is a conflict in American society over the role of government.

Meanwhile, robbing our major governmental health insurance programs, Medicaid and Medicare, through up-coding, unnecessary expensive services, or just plain fraud has led to huge fines. Tenet paid $300 million, HCA/Columbia $740 million, and Blue Cross of Illinois $140 million for overcharging Medicare and Medicaid. Not long ago there was an outcry that Medicare was so inefficient that it had lost $23 billion in over-payments. Yet someone had to bill Medicare. The blame belongs with the (mostly private) health care providers who were systematically (and often fraudulently) overbilling.

Government does have an appropriate role in many functions and does, in fact, do some things right. The events following the September 11 terrorist attacks may have in fact tempered the lack of trust in government. Suddenly, the American public was looking to government for leadership. And the federal government, with the public's blessing, is actually assuming a function formerly done by the private sector: airport security. Other examples of public sector responsibility accepted by the public are defense, road construction, public safety, public education, and the regulation of essential utilities.

A recent example belying the myth that "private is always better" was the deregulation of the power industry. Many people were hurt by the ensuing chaos in energy prices. Americans found themselves exploited by entrepreneurs who maximized their opportunities for profits in the name of the "free market." The debacle was capped by the Enron disaster and recent revelations about how Enron manipulated energy prices. The same phenomenon, though perhaps not quite as obvious, has been happening to health care in America.

When we look at the administrative costs in health care, the comparison between the public and private sectors is not even close. Though it is hard to generalize on the overhead costs for private-sector health insurance, generally it varies between 9 and 30 percent, about 15 percent on the average. These private insurance costs contribute in a major way to the global administrative cost of health care in America—a cost estimated at about 25 percent by Richard Huber, the ex-CEO of Aetna/US Healthcare. Health economist J.D. Kleinke has drawn attention to an even more egregious overhead cost in the private sector: the 50,000 health insurance brokers, or "parasitic middlemen." He estimates they collect commissions that range from 3 to 20 percent of the total cost of insurance plans, adding hundreds of billions of dollars to premium costs.[12]

In contrast, Medicare's overhead is only between two and three percent, and Medicaid (though it varies from state to state) only spends about five or six percent. Some hospital administrators would argue that the bureaucratic regulations put on providers by Medicare actually make their overheads much higher, but many of these same administrators will agree that in the past decade the bureaucratic demands from the private sector (HMOs, etc.) have been just as onerous, if not more.

I queried Thomas Scully, the administrator of the Center for Medicare and Medicaid Services (CMS), about why, at a hearing in October 2001, he had scoffed at the comparative (private vs. Medicare) overhead issue. His reply, via e-mail:

> *"Many make that argument—but I don't agree. We are a blind check-writing machine with two percent overhead. A well-run private insurer has 10-12 percent overhead but has far more understanding of its providers and of patient behavior. The program payments are far less efficiently tracked and targeted...Good insurers are far better at spending money and incentivizing good behavior."*[13]

I assume Mr. Scully was referring to the issue of how money is spent. But there is a huge difference between 2 percent and 10 to12 percent. I suspect that if Medicare, with its economies of scale, had even one percent more to spend to assure the money is spent wisely, it could come up to Mr. Scully's standards. As to incentivizing good behavior, we are on different wavelengths. I described to him my experience with insurers in Idaho. Medicare (as of March 2002), through its contractor Pro-West, had helped 27 health clinics in Idaho to set up a computer-generated preventive screening program. This system provides a detailed reminder sheet at each visit for every Medicare patient. In the case of our clinic (we were the first), they spent thousands of dollars to help us set up a database, which also includes every diabetic patient (about 1000). The result has been greatly improved care for our patients.[14]

In contrast, all I hear from Idaho's premier private insurer is episodic advice on the cost of pharmaceuticals and an occasional clinical education piece that I've already read in a medical journal. There are different kinds of incentives, and "government" often is far superior to the private sector when it comes to prevention.

People have a false impression that Medicare has a bloated bureaucracy. The opposite is actually true. Many of the alleged bureaucratic problems with Medicare have come about because of inadequate staffing—partly as a result of employment freezes—at what used to be called the Health Care Financing Administration (HCFA) and is now CMS. As for the much-disparaged thousands of pages of Medicare regulations, I have been in practice for over 30 years and have yet to read (or felt the necessity to read) even one of these pages. I've probably had good advice from the office staff, and I once even had some charts audited by Medicare (I passed).

The "bottom line" for patient care is that money spent on administration, overhead, marketing, inflated CEO salaries, and corporate profits is money that cannot be spent on patient care. On this "bottom line"—the Veterans Administration notwith-standing, it's a very specialized example—most government programs, including Medicare and Medicaid, far outperform their private counterparts. Moreover, government programs, unlike the private sector, cannot select out the enrollees to avoid the poor, the sick, or the expensive cases.

Government can be ponderous and slow, but at least people have the opportunity to change what they feel is unfair or wrong through the ballot box or by applying public pressure. In contrast, patients have little or no ability to influence the policies of such investor-owned giants such as United Health Care or Aetna, especially in our current situation where it is primarily employers who purchase the insurance for health care. And unfortunately, America's current political system gives corporate lobbyists an advantage over the public in influencing government policy decisions.

Myth #5: Medicare Is Going Broke

MEDICARE IS GOING BROKE. I testified about Medicare before a House subcommittee in Washington in 1994 as part of an "expert" panel. I was reflecting on the future of Medicare from the point of view of the National Rural Health Association. Each Republican on the subcommittee made a point of asking each

panelist—I'm sure for the record—whether we thought
Medicare, if unchanged, was in danger of running out of money.
It reminded me of a lawyer trying to make a point for a jury.
"Medicare in Crisis" is a political game, which has been going on
for many years. Obviously, changes will always have to be
made—and have been made as necessary in the past—to keep
Medicare solvent. Some of the bluster evaporated from the
rhetoric when, after the Balanced Budget Amendment (BBA) of
1997, the costs of Medicare in 1999 actually *decreased* by two
percent. Suddenly, Medicare's solvency got pushed forward by a
few decades. And in 2002, the General Accounting Office, much
to the chagrin of some Republicans, extended the solvency date
of Medicare to 2030.

The real political agenda behind the "crisis" has been, and
continues to be, the privatization, or even the dismantling, of
Medicare. The forces of privatization keep alive the myth of
"Medicare going broke" for the express purpose of scaring the
American people into believing that Medicare should be "saved"
by privatization.

Times have changed since Medicare began in 1965. Although
Medicare benefits have evolved somewhat, such as new added
benefits to cover more preventive measures and (more recently)
Alzheimer's disease, a growing elderly population and new
technologies have made the program much more costly. The
demographic bubble of the aging "baby boomers" will present a
new challenge when this group starts to turn 65 in 2011.

Medicare's current major gap, outpatient pharmaceutical
coverage, is a hotly debated political and economic issue that
needs resolution. There were essentially no expensive drugs in
1965. Today, pharmaceutical costs are about to surpass physician
costs as the second-highest category (after hospital costs)
in health care spending, but Medicare still does not pay for
outpatient drugs. Yet Medicare beneficiaries are the major users
of pharmaceuticals, accounting for 42 percent of all drug sales in
the U.S. The system will adjust, but Medicare is not about to go
under. Meanwhile, many seniors experience great hardship in
order to be able to buy their medications.

Interestingly enough, overall medical costs were steadily going up when Medicare spending decreased two percent in 1999. Perhaps some of the BBA changes that caused this drop were Draconian (such as with home health and hospitals). But the savings for Medicare indicated a considerable amount of "working the system," even fraud. And the drop in Medicare costs illustrates that system changes that control costs are possible. Subsequent adjustments in Medicare that corrected some of the overly zealous sections of the BBA illustrate how our political system can be flexible. The ability of the system to respond to needs is evidence that Medicare is not broken but can be changed or fixed without discarding the whole program. Even the latest crisis, a flawed-formula cut of 5.4 percent in Medicare physician payments, can be resolved.

Medicare beneficiaries are overwhelmingly supportive of Medicare. Study after study shows that people want Medicare improved and expanded, not privatized or dismantled. Yet Republicans and a few Democrats, like Senator John Breaux (D-Louisiana), have sought to privatize Medicare. Perhaps they are acting out of a difference in philosophy (a dislike of public programs). Or maybe their actions are influenced by the advice of lobbyists for special-interest groups that see profits to be made in dismantling Medicare.

These same interest groups are responsible for the myth that a privatized Medicare, or Medicare+Choice, will offer more choice, while the opposite is true. I have a long-time elderly patient who for years had been followed by a certain ear, nose and throat (ENT) physician for his ear problem. Yet when my patient joined a Medicare HMO (one of the Blues' *Mediwonder* plans, touted by advertisements with smiling seniors on the golf course), he could no longer see the ENT doctor who did surgery on his ear. He had to go to a new specialist. More choice? The original Medicare offers full choice of any health care provider. Directing Medicare towards managed care (and choice of plans) has only diminished *real* choice.

Myth #6: We Can't Afford Universal Coverage

AMERICA CAN'T AFFORD UNIVERSAL coverage. This myth gets reinforcement from those who see personal (or corporate) advantages for continuing the status quo with its opportunities for profits. It plays to the fears of those who feel they already have fairly adequate health care coverage. Examples of these relatively well-off people are certain union groups and retirees. The hypothesis is that if everyone is to be covered, then people who now have fairly good coverage will have to give up or sacrifice some benefits so that there will be enough money to include everyone.

Most Americans do not realize that (a) every other industrialized developed country assures coverage for everyone and (b) despite covering everyone, they spend considerably less than we do for health care. The U.S. spends about twice as much per capita than most industrialized countries. In 1998, the U.S. per capita spending for health care was about $4200, compared to $2800 in Switzerland (the next highest), $2400 in Germany (third most expensive), $2300 in Canada, and $1400 in the United Kingdom.[15] As a percent of GDP, in 1998 health care spending represented 13.6 percent of our GDP, compared with 10.6 percent for Germany, 9.5 percent in Canada, and 6.7 percent in the United Kingdom.[16]

These comparative figures sometimes trigger the Alpha Myth (discussed above) that "America has the best health care system in the world," and, of course, the assertion that, "We wouldn't want the type of inferior health care they have in those other countries." This judgment reflects our insularity and ignorance of what actually happens in the other countries. None of the other systems is perfect, and all of them have their problems and their critics, just as we have problems and critics in the U.S. But they do spend a lot less to cover everybody, and their health outcomes are better than ours. Much of the disinformation about other health systems has been disseminated purposefully by organizations such as the AMA.

As for people who live in those other countries (e.g., Canada and England), they are often appalled when they hear about how health care works in the U.S. The great majority of them wouldn't even consider switching their systems for ours. Of course, there are the exceptions. Access to advanced technology in the U.S. is a draw to some rich foreigners who come to famous U.S. clinics for their care. Ironically, a great number of Americans who live right here cannot partake of that technology because they can't afford it.

We have such a frightfully wasteful and fragmented health system in the U.S.—such a complex patchwork of illogical, perverse incentives—that it will be difficult to make the system affordable unless we do basic and significant reform. As discussed above, the estimates vary, but the overall administrative costs of the U.S. system are about 25 to 30 percent. Current estimates of that cost in California, with its terminally developed managed-care systems, run much higher. Tinkering incrementally with the current system, inventing new financial mechanisms such as refundable tax credits, supplemental insurance for all, or medical savings accounts, will only make the system more complex and more wasteful administratively.

What if we had a system such as an improved Medicare for All, with everyone automatically included? It would be not only fair and just, but would also allow huge administrative savings, at the very least over 50 percent. Health economist Donald Light points out that the overhead of the American health care system is "about three times the overhead in countries with private care but universal access, such as Germany, Japan, and The Netherlands."[17] Those savings alone, about $200 billion in 2002, would easily cover the costs of insuring every person in America. After all, we already pay for the uninsured in one way or another. Without spending one more penny as a nation, we could go a long way toward eliminating the suffering, the pain and the worry that come from being uninsured or underinsured.

Study after study has shown that universal coverage with a simplified administrative structure, like national health insurance with everyone in "one risk pool," would actually cost us less while including everybody. From the Congressional Budget Office and General Accounting Office studies of the early '90s to the more recent state-by-state studies, the single-payer approach has consistently been shown to save money. The most recent studies were done as a part of the state health planning grants funded by the Health Resources Service Administration (HRSA). They showed overall savings of more than 5 percent in both Vermont and California with a single-payer plan that included universal coverage. This type of system with "one risk pool" may be the *only* affordable solution.

What percentage of a country's GDP is appropriate to spend on health care is a whole other (and related) philosophic question. From the viewpoint of corporate America, it seems obscene (and uncompetitive) that General Motors spends nearly $3000 for employee health care for every car it produces. But that figure helps bring home the point about perverse incentives. We should be looking at health care from the perspective of the nation as a whole, not just from the point of view of the health care industry. We need to consider breaking the perverse link between employment and health insurance, a link which is not only an accident and unique to America but is also actually hurting U.S. industry by making it less competitive in a world market. The question of how much of our country's GDP we should be spending on health care will be discussed more fully in Chapter 11.

Myth #7: Americans Don't Want "Rationing" of Health Care

AMERICANS WILL NOT ACCEPT *health care "rationing" like they have in other countries.* "Rationing" is a catchword—like "socialized medicine"—that triggers a series of negative gut reactions. Similar to the way Republicans and Democrats have used the words "death tax" and "estate tax" to mean the same thing, people will argue about whether the time one waits to get a certain procedure done or see a particular doctor should be called "rationing" or "waiting time."

But we already have "rationing" or "waiting times" in America. Maybe Americans don't wait as long to get an MRI or a cardiac catheterization because we have an excess capacity for those kinds of expensive procedures. But how long do we Americans have to wait to get an appointment with an ophthalmologist, an orthopedist, or a lung doctor? My elderly aunt in Chicago who needed a hip replacement had to wait three months to see the doctor she wanted. And the chief resident of a Johns Hopkins residency program had to wait almost three months for an appointment with a lung specialist. How long would you have to wait to get a physical exam with your family physician? When I asked that question of my HMO in Boston a few years ago, I was told six months. Rationing or waiting time?

How about the uninsured? I have a patient who has been waiting several years to have her gallbladder taken out. If she had shown up in the emergency room with a "hot" gallbladder and a temperature of 102, she would have had it taken out immediately, no questions asked. Of course, as a result, she might have needed to make payments to a collection agency for the next 10 years. But what if her attack hadn't been acute, and her pain and nausea just came back now and then, as is the case with my patient? She'd wait until she became eligible for Medicare at age 65 to get her surgery. I had another uninsured patient with a painful prolapsed uterus who waited about two years (until she got Medicare) to get treated. Multiply these patients by a few million to get an idea of the magnitude of the problem we Americans already have with "rationing."

The definition of U.S.-style rationing is: (a) If you can afford it, you can get it; (b) If you can't afford it, you either can't or won't get it unless (c) it's a dire emergency and (d) you're lucky enough to catch the problem in time and survive.

Myth #8: We Don't Want Socialized Medicine Like in Canada

CANADA'S HEALTH CARE SYSTEM is terrible and failing. Americans largely dismiss the Canadian system as not worth looking at because the American media campaigns to discredit Canada have been so effective. The U.S. has a high degree of ignorance about the Canadian system. Even some of my friends who are actively working in health care look down on it. "We don't want Canadian-style health care in America," they say. Often we hear such truisms as, "There are more MRI machines in Houston than there are in all of Canada." Maybe Houston should have fewer.

When I talk about health care reform, I frequently get an array of Canada-bashing type questions—except from the Canadians, who often come up after the session to praise their system and scratch their heads over why the U.S. system is so bad. Canadians are outraged at the hatchet jobs that certain U.S. interest groups (like the AMA and the pharmaceutical industry) have done on the Canadian system. The great majority of Canadians are fiercely proud of their health care system (called medicare with a small "m"). They would not even remotely consider changing it for the American system, which many of them (as well as many Europeans) regard as barbaric.

The Canadian health system has its problems, mostly originating from years of underfunding when a conservative government was in power. There are some waiting times for non-emergency services. But personal communications and studies being done indicate that these waiting times are nowhere near as long or onerous as the critics of the Canadian system (who call them "rationing") claim. But the Canadians do have universal coverage with a single-payer system for each province. No one worries about going without needed care or about going bankrupt should he/she have a serious illness. And it's *not* socialized medicine, as the detracting propagandists would have us believe. The delivery system is overwhelmingly private. We have much to learn from Canada.[18] The Canadian system will be discussed further in Chapter 10.

Myth #9: The Insured Pay More to Help Cover the Costs of the Uninsured

THE INSURED ARE SUBSIDIZING the care of the uninsured. This used to be true, but it's often the opposite today. This myth, and its opposing counterpart, demonstrates why universal coverage with "one risk pool" would be fairer. The "cost-shifting" of yesterday, which was unfair in itself, isn't so simple anymore. Today everybody pays more, but because of the practice of "charge inflation"—jacking up prices so they can be discounted for health plans—the uninsured and people with individual insurance are now substantially subsidizing the care of those with group insurance plans. "Hospitals, clinics, labs and physicians charge individuals [including the uninsured] about four to five times as much as their regular negotiated fees with the plans and insurers. [And] insurance companies charge [individuals] much higher premiums for less coverage on the argument that they are at serious risk when they insure one person at a time."[19]

The groups most adversely affected by this practice are Hispanics (the ethnic group with the highest rate of uninsurance, 32 percent in 2000) and immigrants. These practices have been documented by Consejo de Latinos Unidos, and they are suing Tenet in a class-action suit for ethnic discrimination.[20]

The largest subsidy to the insured (and not enjoyed by the uninsured) comes through the tax-free insurance payments made by employers for employee health insurance. This federal subsidy for those with employment-based health insurance amounted to about $140 billion in 2001, or approximately 10 percent of total health care spending. But everyone pays taxes, so the taxes paid by the uninsured, as well as the self-insured, go to pay for health insurance for those with employer-based plans.

The discounts that the managed-care plans have negotiated with hospitals and physician groups mean that the uninsured (and the sheiks) are often the only ones who are now paying full "retail" price.

Of course, some of the uninsured cannot afford to pay, but many do—usually over time and with interest added. On top of being charged several times what the insured are billed, many of the uninsured must also endure the humiliation of being dunned by a collection agency. The poor uninsured person winds up with extra charges and hassles from a collection agency, while the hospital ends up collecting more (even at one-third of the amount billed) from the uninsured person than they would have received from a health plan.

A fall 2000 article[21] in *Health Affairs*, "Gouging the Medically Uninsured: A Tale of Two Bills," describes how the author, who was insured, and her neighbor, who wasn't, paid for their hernia repairs. The uninsured neighbor wound up paying his surgeon (and the hospital) about twice as much for the surgery as did the author, whose HMO had negotiated discount prices with the hospital and physician. I have a low-income uninsured patient, a musician in his forties, who was billed full price (about $2500) for his hernia repair. He's now paying off his bill to a collection agency—principal plus interest. No wonder the 2000 WHO report ranked the U.S. health care system 54th in the world in "fairness."

The fact that the uninsured, who must fend for themselves in buying health care, actually pay more for their care than the insured has great relevance to some of the current proposals now being offered to "reduce the number" of uninsured Americans. Proposals for premium support (as through vouchers) or refundable tax credits would yield a very poor value in today's health care market. Even with generous premium support or tax credits, a person or family seeking insurance coverage in the individual market would still find it unaffordable, especially if there should be a preexisting condition. A recent analysis of the individual insurance market by the Kaiser Family Foundation showed a bleak picture of that market. For example, 35 percent of people applying for insurance were just turned down cold.[22]

Myth #10: Universal Coverage Will Overburden Our System

WE DON'T HAVE THE resources to handle the increased demand for services that would result from universal coverage. The assumption is that if we were to "open the floodgates," the system would be overwhelmed by the pent-up demands for health care from people who were formerly uninsured. In fact, this myth points out the woeful inadequacy of our current system for taking care of the uninsured. The myth also reveals two major faults of our present system: (a) the undersupply of primary care providers compared with the relative oversupply (there are exceptions) of specialists, and (b) the geographic maldistribution of our health care services. Both of these shortcomings are evidence of the market's failure to work for health care.

If the millions of Americans who delay care because they're afraid of the cost came in earlier, it would take stress *off* of the system. Clinicians all appreciate how much less time and effort it takes to care for people who are well compared to the time demands and resource-consuming hassles that accompany medical catastrophes. Yes, there would be a backlog of "catch-up" work that would need to be addressed. But the later we start to deal with the fruits of our neglect, the harder it will be to catch up. There's no doubt that the system needs to change. It must be more responsive to real health care needs, not just the whim of "the market." We have to make it more efficient. And in the reorganization of the system, first priority needs to go to patients and their needs.

Universal coverage should lead to the more appropriate use of emergency rooms (ERs) once people have improved access to primary care. ERs would be used for true emergencies, instead of the host of non-emergency cases that now clog their corridors. We'll have to find ingenious ways to meet an initial excess demand in a timely manner. We have a sufficient number of health care providers—even nurses, if we count all the nurses who now do administrative duties or who have left nursing out of frustration over adverse working conditions.

The possible solutions include: (a) more efficient use of primary care providers (with decreased administrative tasks, they should be able to do more patient care); (b) shifting of some specialist time into primary care; (c) increased use of mid-level clinicians, such as nurse practitioners and physician assistants; and (d) extra rewards for doing primary care in areas that are medically underserved. Eventually, when the "delayed care backlog" is caught up, the excess utilization should even out. The controversial issue of whether Americans are overutilizers of care will be discussed more fully in Chapter 2.

Myth #11: Costs of "Research and Development" Drive Our Higher Drug Prices

DRUG PRICES ARE HIGHER in the U.S. because our pharmaceutical industry spends billions of dollars on research and development.

All the evidence shows this assertion to be a myth, a figment of creative accounting. The drug companies have the highest profit margin of all American corporations. Their profits as a percent of sales run about 19 percent, compared to a median of about 5 percent for all the Fortune 500 companies.[23] Data from the drug companies' annual reports show that they spend almost three times as much on marketing and administrative costs as they spend on research and development (R&D)[24]—a discrepancy totally ignored in a July 2002 HHS report linking innovation in drug development to the freedom from government controls.[25]

© Tribune Media Services, Inc. All Rights Reserved. Reprinted with permission.

The drug companies claim that it costs them over $800 million (a recent number, it used to be only $500 million) to bring a new drug to market. This number is grossly exaggerated. Creative accounting—akin to the type used by Enron—has been used to inflate the true costs. They have included such items as "lost-opportunity costs" in doing their calculations. Other experts who have examined the data come up with much lower figures for R&D. Their estimates are closer to $100 million, a huge difference. *Public Citizen* put their estimate of the real number at $110 million (for 2000).[26]

Drug prices are much higher in America than in any other country—about 60 percent higher, on the average, than the prices in Canada and the U.K. Our drug companies claim that the U.S. pharmaceutical industry carries the burden of doing R&D for the rest of the world. Yet the European countries (combined) put out approximately the same number of new drugs a year as we do in America. And our drug industry's R&D gets huge taxpayer subsidies from government-supported drug research done by our National Institutes of Health and American universities.[27]

Our patent laws allow new drugs to become mini-monopolies, with "anything goes" pricing. And, with all of the new drugs produced in America, only a very small percentage are in fact innovative developments. Most are varieties of old drugs, like an extended-release product, developed to extend patent protections. Community needs are given a low priority.

The reason drugs cost more in America than in any other country boils down to one simple factor: the pursuit of maximum profit. The pharmaceutical industry has taken every opportunity, used every ploy, to deceive the American people. To derail efforts at making pharmaceutical benefits an integral part of Medicare, they spent tens of millions of dollars on an advertising campaign ("the bus from Canada") to discredit the Canadian system, and even created a bogus organization, "Citizens for Better Medicare," to try to lend credibility to their efforts. And now they are introducing piecemeal discount card programs in an effort to defuse efforts for more comprehensive change.

Some of the other questionable, and often illegal, ploys used by the pharmaceutical industry include:

- Manipulating patent law to keep cheaper generic products off the market (as with Taxol),[28] or paying off smaller pharmaceutical companies not to manufacture cheaper generic versions of their drugs, as has happened with BuSpar and Hytrin.[29]

- Giving kickbacks to physicians who overcharge Medicare for drugs. TAP Pharmaceuticals paid a record $875 million fine for abuses involving their prostate cancer drug Lupron.

- Price-fixing. In a case involving vitamins, several pharmaceutical companies paid a fine of over $700 million.

- Paying off the "pharmaceutical benefit managers" who are supposed to save money for health care organizations by selecting cheaper drugs. They gave them bonuses for promoting drugs that were not always the most economical.[30]

- The systematic "bribing" of the medical profession and our legislators through an array of questionable but legal activities, from gifts and free lunches to campaign contributions.[31]

- The creation of so-called "Astroturf" grassroots support groups, like "Citizens for a Better Medicare," to give the impression there is popular support for or against a particular issue, such as a prescription benefit as an integral part of Medicare.

In its pursuit of profitability, the pharmaceutical industry is one of the most formidable obstacles to health care reform in America. Spending on their products has been increasing by 15 to 20 percent a year. With pharmaceutical costs about to surpass physician costs, only hospital costs are higher. The pharmaceutical industry enjoys enormous privileges in the form of generous tax benefits and patent protections. They operate without price controls, a unique circumstance among the developed nations of the world. They are performing a superb job in carrying out their mission to maximize stockholder profits, even if it means that millions of elderly Americans must choose between medicines or food.

Marcia Angell, the former editor of the *New England Journal of Medicine*, argues in an editorial that because of the pharmaceutical industry's large taxpayer subsidy, and "because it makes products of vital importance to the public health, it should be accountable not only to its shareholders, but also to society at large."[32]

Myth #12: We Can Get to Universal Coverage Through Incremental Changes

WE CAN GET TO universal coverage through incremental or piecemeal changes. When the overly complex Clinton Plan died in 1994, efforts ceased for a comprehensive solution to help the uninsured. It seems that about every decade or so some momentum builds towards enacting universal coverage. In the past century, these efforts have routinely been beaten back each time—usually by a coalition of well-financed and politically influential interest groups. The traditional opponents of comprehensive change such as national health insurance have been the AMA, the insurance industry, the pharmaceutical industry, and certain other business interests. After the reform debacle of 1994, politicians looked at comprehensive change with the deference owed a third rail. Popular wisdom dictated that the only politically safe route to take in efforts at health care reform was the path of "incremental" change.

What have the incremental efforts of the past decade brought us? We've seen an increase of about five million in the number of uninsured. After a brief period of relative cost containment thanks to the temporary effects of managed care and the denial of care to millions, we once again have double-digit inflation annually in the cost of health insurance. And despite an ambitious (and, in some states, relatively successful) Children's Health

Insurance Program, the number of uninsured children remains only minimally reduced, still at about nine million.

And now, with a seemingly reborn interest in increasing health insurance coverage, there is a plethora of ideas and proposals that have been accompanied by a lot of talk but so far not much action. They use the word "universal" fleetingly but really seem to mean "incremental." Foundations and the federal government (through HRSA) are paying millions of dollars to consultants and planners to come up with bold new ideas for providing health care coverage for more Americans. Many of the proposals, as noted above, are not really about "universal" coverage. Even in their broadest implementation, most of the plans leave millions of Americans uncovered. Instead of truly being bold, they defer to the fickle god of "political reality."

Reflecting our present quagmire of health insurance options, the new proposals postulate a complex and confusing array of approaches. Using the expansion of Medicaid and CHIP as an initial step, they propose a mix of refundable tax credits, federal subsidies, medical savings accounts, vouchers, employer-defined contributions, supplemental insurance policies to cover drugs or items that primary insurance doesn't cover, and buying cooperatives—among other ideas.

For my patients and millions of other Americans like them, the complexity of many of these proposals makes them pipe dreams. They are simply too complex and costly for the average near-poor family without health insurance, as well as for the growing millions who are inadequately insured. Each little part of these "incremental" or "piecemeal" approaches would likely help a limited number of people. But the added complexity will only serve to raise the overall administrative costs. And more people (perhaps different ones) will fall between the ever-enlarging cracks in the system. Meanwhile, the complexity enables the corporate groups with the smartest consultants and lawyers to continue to game the system.

In an essay looking at universal coverage in the U.S. from a historical perspective, Karen Davis, president of the Commonwealth Fund, remarks that "incremental changes that expand coverage but do not change the organization and delivery of services have fared better than more sweeping health care reform proposals that would have a substantial impact on the economic interests of health care providers and insurers."[33] Comprehensive change is difficult, yet "incremental" approaches have been slow and frustrating. Speaking of the uninsured in 1998, Drew Altman, president of the Kaiser Family Foundation, said, "We have been making some progress with the small incremental reforms, but it's like shoveling sand against the tide."

What about expansion of the federal programs, Medicare, Medicaid, and CHIP? The Medicaid and/or CHIP route has been the "incremental" path that most states have chosen to pursue. These approaches offer generous matching funds from Washington, up to 80 percent in the case of CHIP. Some states, such as Rhode Island, have included people up to 400 percent of the poverty level in the programs. Several states are starting to cover parents of CHIP beneficiaries. Yet most states have been much less generous. They see Medicaid and CHIP, even with the federal match, as an increasingly onerous drain on their state budgets.

States like Oregon and Minnesota have been innovative in their program design but, at least in the case of Oregon, the results have been far from adequate. The August 1, 2001, Portland *Oregonian* reported a study which showed that 43 percent of the people covered by the Oregon Health Plan, the state's medical safety net for the poor, leave the plan within a year. They left largely because they earned just a little too much to qualify, but they still couldn't afford private insurance. A case example from our practice illustrates the dilemma:

> *Eighteen-year-old Mindy seriously injured her shoulder at work 10 months ago. She required surgery and Workmen's Compensation paid for it. Four months later, she reinjured the shoulder and was seen at the ER. The ER physician told her to follow up with a bone specialist, but she didn't since she couldn't afford it. Instead, she came into our health center two months later with a badly deformed shoulder. We determined that she*

*would qualify for CHIP, so we arranged an appointment
with a bone specialist. Unfortunately, CHIP expires at age
19 and she turned 19 two days later, so she lost her insurance coverage and is once again unable to pay for care.*

Medicaid theoretically has an excellent benefit package
though it varies widely from state to state, as do the eligibility
requirements. It also has nearly no co-pays, but as it exists
today, Medicaid is far from ideal. It reimburses poorly. It's often
difficult to find providers who will take patients with Medicaid,
especially for dental services. Each state program is at the mercy
of state budget-setters on a year-to-year basis. And Medicaid has
a stigma attached to it, the aura of welfare. A recent study in
the *American Journal of Public Health* on problems with access
to dental care for Medicaid-insured children illustrates this
phenomenon. Summarizing the results of that study:

> *"Negative experiences with the dental care system
> discouraged many caregivers...from obtaining dental
> services for their...children. ...Caregivers who success-
> fully negotiated [the many logistic] barriers felt that
> they encountered additional barriers in the dental care
> setting, including long waiting times and judgmental,
> disrespectful, and discriminatory behavior from staff
> and providers because of their race and public assistance
> status."*[34]

Medicaid's worst problem is perhaps its impermanence for
individuals. Because of Medicaid's eligibility requirements,
many people have only transient coverage. They can get easily
dropped from the program. This fickle nature of Medicaid
especially affects the working near-poor, many of whom are
without insurance today. Yet manipulating Medicaid and/or
CHIP, with or without federal waivers, is by far the simplest
means of doing "incremental" change in a state. Arizona used
the Medicaid expansion tactic in 2000 by deciding to provide
Medicaid coverage for all people up to 100 percent of poverty.

However, with the economic recession, all Medicaid approaches, including Arizona's, are endangered.

In a recent article about Medicaid, Sara Rosenbaum explores its precarious current situation.[35] Tight state budgets and the newly available waivers threaten to trim benefits for people with Medicaid. Only a short while ago, Medicaid and CHIP were "the low-lying fruit" for planners looking at ways to expand coverage. No more.

One peculiar aspect of Medicaid that has pretty much escaped scrutiny is its relation to nursing homes. As the major payer for nursing home services (an irrationality of its role—why shouldn't Medicare be the payer?), Medicaid expenses for nursing homes have been fairly untouchable. Since nursing home reimbursements represent about half of Medicaid costs, states are fairly hamstrung when it comes to cutting services. It has become a reverse "lifeboat" paradigm: dump the women and children first. Meanwhile, the nursing homes are incredibly squeezed and care is inadequate. A government study released in February 2002 reported that over 90 percent of U.S. nursing homes lacked adequate staffing.[36] Registered nurse positions were found to be staffed at barely over half the recommended level.

The Commonwealth Fund's 2000 proposal for (near) universal coverage—again, the play on words—envisages a great expansion of Medicaid to include all low-income people. And it puts high-risk people into Medicare. The healthy and relatively wealthy would be left for the private sector. It would be far from universal, do nothing to decrease administrative costs or complexity, and give a huge gift to the insurance industry. Moreover, it would further institutionalize a multi-tiered health care system in the U.S.

As Uwe Reinhardt, the Princeton health economist, said about "incremental" reforms in 1999, "The problem lies in the self-destruct mechanism inherent in the very idea of incrementalism. Even Mother Theresa probably could not make incrementalism work any better. It has been thus and it always will be thus."[37]

We are seeing a variety of efforts toward incremental change today. Some, like myself, who advocate for comprehensive change, nonetheless pursue some of the incremental efforts *du jour,* such as follow-up care for women who are found to have breast cancer, because our patients are in need. Although they see the need, others have given up on trying to get comprehensive change. For them, incremental changes appear to be the only direction feasible in today's political climate. These well-intentioned people pursuing the route of noncomprehensive incremental change are pragmatists, as I am also on certain days. Many of them have become discouraged and have lost faith, at least temporarily.

The vested interests may have more cynical reasons for encouraging incremental change. They appreciate that such limited tweaking of the system will basically maintain the status quo and thereby assure the present balance of power and profits. The more cynical among them also may be encouraging the incremental path because it gives the appearance of doing *something* while avoiding the more fundamental questions. It's uncertain how long such stopgap measures such as discount coupons for drugs or reinsurance for inadequate insurance will forestall a real revolution in health care financing, a grassroots uprising that will eventually demand that health care be a right, and not a privilege, in the U.S.

Are there incremental-type changes that can lead to a just system of universal coverage? Probably yes. The types of progressive or "sequential" incremental change that could lead to universal coverage could be measures that are all-inclusive of a specific age group of our population. For example, we could put all children, or all people aged 55–64, in an expanded Medicare as a first step. Similarly, a state-by-state strategy (as a first step) could also work as it did in Canada, but it would be much more difficult because of the legal hurdles that would have to be overcome. At least these kinds of approaches would obviate the gaming of the system that excludes the sick and the poor.

Then there is the incremental approach proposed in April 2002 by the American College of Physicians–American Society of Internal Medicine. It meets the criterion of progressively reaching the goal of universal coverage (everyone included). They outline how universal coverage could be reached in stages over seven years. But the proposal's framework is built upon expansion of Medicaid and CHIP with the addition of premium support. Although they admit they are dealing exclusively with the issue of "coverage," they are skirting the issue of affordability. Instead of addressing the failures, inefficiencies, and inequities of our current fragmented system, they are taking the approach of "throwing money at the system"—feeding the monster. Given the current political climate and the reality of our political institutions, I doubt their brand of "incremental" has a better chance of being adopted than a pure single-payer approach.

Although it's uncertain how long the economy will continue to suffer, the current worsening economic situation bodes poorly for the success of incremental approaches. With increasing unemployment, a growing number of uninsured, rapidly rising health care costs, and a diminishing ability to fund government-financed "safety-net" programs like Medicaid, we need a more comprehensive solution. As David Broder said in an op-ed piece in the *Washington Post*, "It is...clear that tinkering around the edges cannot, for long, withstand the adverse trends that are at work, let alone reverse them."[38]

Myth #13: Americans Won't Accept Single-Payer Universal Coverage

AMERICANS WILL NEVER ACCEPT a single-payer system. This myth, which will be explored in more detail in Chapters 14 and 15, is a particularly critical point for the vested interests. The special-interest groups that promote this myth take every opportunity to exclude single-payer advocates from discussions of health care reform. They assert that we must have a "pluralistic" approach to health care reform, thereby assuring their hegemony. The American people, who have been exposed only to the rhetoric of the vested interests, have not had the opportunity to form any thoughtful consensus on the single-payer approach. The merchants of misinformation and myth have been successful at hawking a line of philosophic incompatibility to discredit the single-payer approach—"we hate government, we don't want socialized medicine."

Columnist Molly Ivins noted: "Every time we start to get serious about reform, the right wing starts screaming, 'Socialized medicine, socialized medicine.' And then we're all supposed to run screaming with horror."[39] Ivins goes on to endorse the type of solution that every other industrialized country has embraced: "Universal health insurance, a single-payer system." Single payer is not "socialized medicine," nor does it need to be "big government."

Unfortunately, the term "single payer" is oversimplified. Even advocates for universal coverage disagree on the use of the term. But in general, "single payer" identifies an approach based on "one risk pool" with everyone included, like national health insurance. A summary of the principles that comprise the "single-payer" with "one risk pool" type of solution is found at the end of the Introduction to this book.

Can you imagine what a national health insurance system with group (meaning, every American) clout could do in negotiating discounts in drug prices? If I were the pharmaceutical industry, I'd worry—and they do. Their $38 billion in profits in 2000 could be cut in half, although there are reasonable theories that argue that increased sales under a program of national health insurance would offset the losses from lower prices. It's not hard to wonder why they spend so many millions on lobbying, campaign contributions, and expensive advertising campaigns. As for the health insurance industry, they would be fighting for their very existence.

How about the AMA? As a physician, I'm ashamed of them. They've forgotten the primary mission of physicians as caregivers. As an organization, the AMA has lost touch with reality. They have little appreciation for what it means to be uninsured. Nor do they know how little it really matters to be able to exercise "personal responsibility" in the chaotic, fragmented, and illogical health care environment that exists in America today.

Americans overwhelmingly support universal coverage, yet they are largely doubtful that we can accomplish the goal. Their doubt is the result of a purposeful campaign of misinformation and disinformation to "keep America clueless." The mythology works to create the sense that universal coverage with a single-payer type system is a pipe dream, not to be considered seriously. For the moment, it's politically difficult to promote the single-payer approach, like Medicare for All or national health insurance. But the winds of politics can change in the blink of an eye.

Though economic conditions in America can change quickly, the near future appears to be bringing deterioration in the status of both the uninsured and the insured. America is facing the danger of a "health care meltdown" that will threaten the well-being of middle-class America. Many more middle-class Americans will be hurting. Grassroots indignation and unrest could ensue, with a demand for real change in how we finance health care in this country. In 2000, a ballot initiative for single-payer type universal coverage just barely missed passage (48 percent to 52 percent) in Massachusetts.

How long can the special interests maintain the myths? More importantly, how much longer will the American people tolerate having their own health care needs kept subservient to the self-serving goals of the special-interest groups? Only as long as the American people can be kept clueless.

Unfortunately, the myths have helped to maintain and nurture the "monster" that our American health care system has become. The following two chapters explore this "monster."

Summary of Key Points

- The American people have been led to believe a series of myths about our health care system, myths that impede change.

- "The market" has been a failure for health care in America. Health care is not a commodity like fast food or automobiles.

- For health care, the public sector in fact has a much lower overhead than the private sector.

- There is a better way: universal coverage with "one risk pool."

- Health care for all *is* affordable, but will require basic reforms of our current crazy, dysfunctional system.

- Incremental approaches have not led to significant change in our system but have only delayed the implementation of real change.

- "One risk pool" with everybody in—and nobody out—is *not* socialized medicine.

If not called for in 10 days P.M. return to
Dr. E. SMITH, Normal, Ills.

Chapter 2

America's Health Care:
The Monster We Have Created

"...As soon as I started to learn about health care and health insurance, I was so struck by the craziness of the system and how unjust it is and how it makes no sense."
— Health policy expert Rima Cohen[1]

The 72-year-old woman was overweight and had diabetes. She also had a stuffy nose and railroad insurance that covered the cost of prescriptions not covered by Medicare. Instead of buying an inexpensive over-the-counter medication, she asked that I prescribe a $90 a month non-sedating kind of antihistamine. "My insurance pays for it," she said, "I don't care what it costs."

Another woman, 64 years old, has diabetes and high blood pressure. She misses her appointments and tells me that she takes her medicines only two or three times a week because, "Doc, that's all I can afford." Her blood sugar is 300 (normal being about 100) and her blood pressure 160/110 (normal being less than 140/90).

QUITE POSSIBLY FRANZ KAFKA and Dr. Frankenstein were collaborators in the design of our American health care system, and they carried out their work with grant funding from the Alfred Hitchcock Foundation. Or so it seems. The United States has always had an aversion to health planning ("socialism!"), but our love of laissez-faire "free-market" principles has helped create a "monster" of a health care system, or more correctly stated, nonsystem. And as we struggle with the difficulty of implementing change in America, we are seeing our already deficient health system get even worse. Perhaps Mr. Kafka has returned as the CEO of an HMO.

"My insurance covers MRIs, doc. So I'd like to have one." How often have we physicians heard this request, or others like it for a variety of tests, procedures, or referrals? "I've got a pain in my knee. I need a referral to a bone doctor." I recently saw a 60-year-old man with heart disease who saw an ad for the blood thinner Plavix on TV. He asked me to prescribe it for him (at $110 a month) instead of the daily aspirin he was taking—even though he wouldn't quit smoking. These requests often come without any discussion. I've had patients (insured, of course) request total body CAT scans to help tell them why they have some vague aches and pains—again, even before discussing the symptoms. Meanwhile, those very tests are being marketed to the public— no doctor's referral necessary.

On the other hand, the uninsured patients want as little done as possible. "Please, doc, no lab tests today. I can't afford them." But it's amazing what "catch-up" medical work gets done when someone gets health insurance or turns 65 and qualifies for Medicare. Suddenly the gallbladder that's been acting up off and on for eight years is taken out, the diagnostic tests for angina are done. Perhaps most frustrating for me as a physician are the chronic disease patients who won't return for needed follow-ups because they can't afford the visits. These are the people with poorly controlled hypertension, diabetes, or heart disease, who "live with" their ailments. Even at our community health center, which has a (now) $10 "nominal" fee for a visit, many won't come back until they're out of medications—or worse.

There's a disconnect here. Although these are a few simple examples of the paradoxes and inequities in our system, health care in America, as it has evolved in a haphazard way, is really extremely complicated and full of contradictions, inefficiencies, and chaos. A "health care hodgepodge," as the *Des Moines Register* editorial board termed it in a recent editorial piece.[2] If we were to look at our system from the outside, we could easily conclude that, given our generous resources as the richest country in the world, we couldn't have designed a more dysfunctional system if we had tried.

In his recent book, *As Sick as It Gets,*[3] Rudy Mueller, M.D., describes in minute and excruciating detail just how frightful our system has become. He relates how it affects people's daily lives and robs them not only of their money, but also of their dignity. I see the horrors of our nonsystem every day in my own community health center practice. The irrationality, the inhumanity, the greed, the inequity, and even the cruelty are incomprehensible for a nation that wants to believe "we have the best health care system in the world."

It's not that millions of American health care workers, from receptionists to physicians, are not trying to do their best to serve patients with diligence and compassion. I see many good-faith efforts to help people every day. But our broken system puts unnecessary (and often senseless) obstacles in the way of people getting the health care they need. And the self-destructiveness of the system has only accelerated in the past two decades with the transformation of American health care from what was primarily a caring endeavor to a commercial enterprise. Kathleen O'Connor, in her book, *The Buck Stops Nowhere,*[4] demonstrates the perversion of our system in her first chapter on "healthcare's battlefield." She devotes 36 pages of that chapter to the games of financing and "the market" and less than two pages to "the patient." Our priorities have been turned upside down.

We've created a huge monster. We continue to nourish the monster because powerful financial interest groups, like the pharmaceutical industry, the insurance companies, large employers, and some elements of the medical establishment, know that any real solution could threaten their bottom lines. So they have helped to create a mythology to plant the doubt that Americans who are already insured might lose something if there were to be any real changes.

Thus, we see a series of proposals to "tweak the monster" and make it more complicated and incomprehensible—all to delay the inevitable (real change). And to heck with the patients. They are being enticed to pay more and more of the costs while being lulled to complacency by flowery phraseology such as "more choice," "consumer-directed care," or "personal health accounts." The monster continues to grow, and as it grows, it devours our resources and squelches any good intentions. The monster has many dimensions.

Managed Care vs. Managed Cost: "Crazy Making"

MUCH HAS BEEN WRITTEN and debated on the experience with "managed care" in America, a uniquely American experience in "crazy making," especially for *insured* Americans. The response of Americans to a movie like "John Q," which portrays how the managed-care industry "jerks people around" and denies needed care, demonstrates how much health insurers have come to be reviled by the American public—perhaps second only to the tobacco industry.

Managed care itself is basically a sound concept. The alternative, "unmanaged care"—care delivered without regard to scientific evidence, cost, or relevance to the individual or society—is clearly inappropriate. The current trend towards rational "disease management" is a positive aspect of managed care. America's prime example of the old style of managed care, Kaiser Permanente, a not-for-profit group health plan, had, and still has, many favorable qualities. Responding to a recent flawed analysis in the *British Medical Journal*,[5] which compared California's Kaiser Permanente to Britain's National Health System (NHS), health policy expert Kevin Grumbach remarked that, "Within the disorganized and inefficient context of the overall U.S. health care system, Kaiser does stand out as an admirable model of health care integration...."[6]

But managed care in America has gone astray. Its original purpose, as with the old Kaiser model, was to coordinate and improve patient care. However, when the concept was applied to eliminating waste and inefficiencies in the health care system, not a bad end in itself, the whole emphasis changed to "managed cost." The patient focus was lost and became a secondary goal. The result has been more "mangled cared" than "managed care." "The market" and economic interests became the driving force for health care in America. As a local employer explained to me, he had three motivations for embracing managed care: "Cost, cost, and cost." As a result, the insured in America have been "jerked around"—and will continue to be "jerked around"—by insurers and employers if we continue in the direction we appear to be headed.

Movies like "John Q" and the Showtime movie released in May 2002, "Damaged Care," touch a raw nerve with the American public. "Damaged Care" tells the true story of Linda Peeno, M.D., who, as medical director of Humana, was forced to deny care systematically so that profits could be maximized for the corporation. Most people, however, have little appreciation for the abuses of "managed cost" until they (or one of their family members) have a serious illness and a hands-on encounter with the managed-care industry. Many Americans come away from the experience with a total disbelief on just how crazy—and uncaring—our system has become. And as our system heads towards "meltdown," the situation will only get worse, especially for middle-class Americans.

Unrealistic Expectations

FROM "MARCUS WELBY," TO "ER," to media splashes about technological advances such as mechanical hearts and limb replacements, even to the "direct-to-consumer" ads pushing cures for toenail fungus or seasonal allergies, the American public has been led to expect wonders from our health care system. The smiling, athletic people in the HMO ads don't expect to have their claims denied when they show up in the ER without preauthorization. And people expecting to spend an hour discussing their health care concerns with Dr. Welby, Jr., don't realize that Doc Welby is expected to see 28 patients a day.

In all fairness, many of the expectations have the potential to be real, at least technologically. Our technology is wonderful. There have been especially great advances in pharmacology. For example, new drugs have nearly eliminated bleeding stomach ulcers and the need for ulcer surgery. The "statin" drugs provide great promise to prevent heart attacks and strokes. New antidepressants and antipsychotics have provided huge advances in the treatment of mental illness. Many of these advances have led to a substantial decrease in the need for hospitalization.

Meanwhile, there have been equally huge leaps forward in such areas as joint replacements, microsurgical techniques, and diagnostic testing, offering an improved state of well-being for many. Surgical procedures that used to require long hospitalizations are now done in day surgery with much less discomfort and trauma for the patient. Future developments in areas such as gene therapy and even greater miniaturization will create a whole new array of possibilities; e.g., curing diabetes or cancer, or even halting the aging process.

But these expectations have been largely divorced from realistic cost factors or affordability. And prevention has taken a distant back seat to expensive and media-hyped interventions aimed at curing illness or fixing injury. Americans, like our health care industry, think short-term. The new technologies are at times amazing and, of course, usually very expensive. But, after all, if it were available, who wouldn't want the "very best" treatment, especially if it were covered by insurance? If your child were ill, wouldn't you want the treatment with the highest chance of success, even if it cost a bundle?

Pharmaceutical industry dollars and the media attention given to medical and technological advances have changed the culture of how Americans look at health care. Americans have come to "expect the world." Of course, the argument could be made that people *should* be able to "expect the world" even though that might involve foregoing something else or resorting to statewide bake sales to pay the bill. The message from the sellers of health care, and the way physicians used to be taught to practice, has clearly been to ignore cost and do the "very best," though it hasn't always been clear that the "very best" is really best. Although the managed-cost gurus have tried to modify the message, physicians' training (at least in the old days) never talked about "Option #2—use in case of uninsurance."

Interestingly enough, there are rifts among the major health care players on this issue of pursuing the "very best" for patients. The pharmaceutical industry and medical specialists push their expensive and often, but not always, more efficacious options. But the insurance industry and managed-care organizations fight to control costs. So the two sides are sometimes at loggerheads, as with the issue of converting certain expensive antihistamines from prescription-only to over-the-counter (OTC) status. Such a change would help insurers, who don't normally pay for OTC drugs. But it would hurt the pharmaceutical companies because people would balk at paying $80 a month out of pocket for a drug when they could buy an almost equivalent product for a few dollars.

Crazy pricing is a major factor in driving up costs. Historically, providers were able to collect whatever they charged, and this "history" has served to perpetuate a system with excessively high price tags, most notably for specialist care and "procedures." "Thinking" clinicians (i.e., clinicians who use cognitive approaches versus procedural interventions) might get reimbursed $35 for talking to a patient for half an hour about multiple medical problems, but pass a tube to someone's stomach (it can be done in 10 minutes) and the payment can be $900. Illogical, but that's our system. Mostly, we've saddled the system with overpayments, but there are also underpayments, as to clinicians who care for Medicaid and some HMO or Medicare patients. Many physicians now refuse to take on patients with Medicaid and/or Medicare if they have enough full-paying patients. Crazy pricing has been particularly harmful for the uninsured and the underinsured. They are increasingly being forced to chose "Option #2" or "Option #3" (no care).

Instead of "great expectations," a large number of Americans must settle for "small expectations," like a woman we recently saw with a 10-inch mass in her abdomen. She's unable to find a surgeon to take out her tumor because she can't afford $1900 up front. After all, that's the way "the market" works. And that's a major reason why there is a fundamental disconnect between "the market" and health care in America.

Ignorance of the Costs

HEALTH ECONOMIST UWE REINHARDT has politely described the way we price health care in America as "one of the most opaque sectors in the economy."[7] He adds, "Many folks must prefer it that way, or it would not be so." Only recently have there been some efforts to educate caregivers about costs. But there appears to be almost no effort yet to educate patients on this critical issue—thus, keeping the demand unabated for, say, expensive drugs. I don't see prices advertised in the glitzy ads for Sporanox, Nexium, or Claritin. It doesn't state in the direct-to-consumer ads that the treatment for toenail fungus costs $800 per course of therapy, or that the "purple pill" for heartburn will cost $120 a month as opposed to Zantac, which can work just as well for a fraction of the cost. It's to the advantage of the pharmaceutical companies for patients to have little idea what their drugs cost. With inpatient care, the patient may never even see the hospital bill if it's paid for by private insurance. Medicare beneficiaries who do see the bottom line of their bill are blown away by the amount.

Physicians used to be taught to forget the cost. The drug reps never used to discuss cost, and now they usually bring it up when they're trying to show how much cheaper their product is compared to their competitors' (e.g., only $110 a month vs. $130). As for diagnostic tests, we physicians hardly ever think of their cost. We order them and expect the patient to get what we ordered. Also unaware of the costs, the patient usually complies. Both the physician and the patient are then surprised when (and if) they find out that the prenatal ultrasound cost $600 or the echocardiogram cost $1000.

Squeezed by economic pressures, hospitals have started to try to educate their doctors on the relative costs of the drugs they prescribe in the hospital, especially since Medicare now gives a fixed diagnosis-related reimbursement for each hospital patient. And managed-care plans have been highly motivated to try to educate their physicians on drug costs. They have created drug formularies, which make sense in theory, but are based mostly on cost, not efficacy. The formularies often complicate matters for the patient, who may be forced to switch drugs and then suffer unfortunate side effects.

We could do much more to lower costs, such as practicing scientifically based medicine, but it's like combating an epidemic. There is such a strong incentive, as with the pharmaceutical industry and surgical subspecialists, to keep prices—and profits or incomes—high. It will likely require a major change in how we organize health care in America to effect any meaningful change. If we were really to practice scientifically based medicine, the cost savings would be great. We order and do so many unnecessary tests and procedures, and our prescribing patterns are illogical and expensive.

Switching from the individual patient to the macroeconomic scale, ignorance of true costs has created major opportunities for maximizing profits. The insurance companies benefit greatly from playing the "ignorance game," as described in a web article entitled "What your health insurer doesn't want you to know."[8] Manipulation of the system, using its complexity and its financial "opacity," has become the norm for health care in America. Arrangements that unnecessarily increase the cost of health care—beyond administrative costs—are being brought to light. Examples: the high added costs of commissions for insurance brokers, inflated drug costs for products supplied by "pharmaceutical benefit managers," and, now, questionable practices by the middlemen who do the group purchasing of medical supplies for hospitals.

As described in an article in *The New York Times*,[9] two private groups (Premier and Novation), acting as middlemen for about half of America's not-for-profit hospitals, may have been compromising their mission to find the best supplies for hospitals at the lowest prices. It appears that the two buying groups, with purchases of $34 billion in 2001, "are financed not by the hospitals that buy the products but by the companies that sell them." The middlemen have financial ties to medical supply companies that are "both extensive and highly unusual." Buying groups are, in effect, getting paid to buy certain products. The situation illustrates how "the market" in health care has encouraged the development of oligopolies with a concomitant abuse of power. It also shows how an industry managed to escape regulatory oversight, as with Enron, by convincing Congress to exempt them from rules such as the federal anti-kickback laws.

The Paperwork Nightmare

There has been a quantum leap in the past 10 to 15 years in the amount of paperwork required to carry out the daily tasks of health care. Paralleling this growth in paperwork has been a vast expansion in the number of people required to administer our system (see the graph showing the comparative growth of physicians and administrators over the past 30 years).

Growth of Physicians and Administrators, 1970-1998

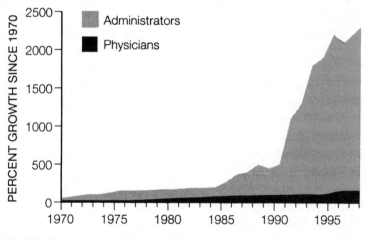

SOURCE: Bureau of Labor Statistics & NCHS

Reprinted with permission.

The fragmentation of insurance coverage, and the accompanying need for establishing eligibility for the various insurance programs, has greatly increased administrative costs and hassles. With respect to eligibility, health policy expert Sherry Glied points out that, "Universal coverage would readily solve all of the problems [with eligibility determination], as would a health insurance system that enrolled everyone automatically and then determined appropriate financing sources."[10] In other words, a single risk pool would simplify our system and require much less paperwork. The more recent increase in paperwork, which claims more and more of providers' time, has come both from the demands of managed-care organizations and from government efforts to stem fraud and abuse.

Some of the most onerous paperwork, sad to say, may be for Medicare, although not so much in the office setting. I pity the poor home health and nursing home workers who must spend three-quarters of their time writing notes about each patient. They cram endless handwritten notes into tiny writing so that the required information fits in the spaces provided. They can't possibly have much time left to care for the patients. Similarly, RNs in hospitals are consumed with filling out forms or completing notes. That's one of the prime reasons why nursing has lost its desirability as a profession. The situation cries out for improvement and simplification.

There's a story about nurses in hospitals being told by supervisors to avoid eye contact with patients when they go into the rooms. If they don't make eye contact, they will spend less time talking to the patient and, presumably, will have more time for their administrative chores.

The Medicare forms for durable medical equipment are complex, often incomprehensible, and take lengthy efforts to complete. If I could think of the number-one reason I would consider quitting the practice of medicine, it would be these forms. For hospitals, Medicare requirements are a burden, requiring extra staff and resources—resources that are diverted from patient care. But the managed-care companies have also done a good job of creating at least an equal burden of tedious paperwork for hospitals and other providers. Case in point: there's a story about Michael Dukakis visiting a large hospital in Vancouver, B.C., and asking to see their administrative wing. When he was shown two small rooms and told that was their entire billing department, he was flabbergasted. There are some things we could learn from Canada, even if the AMA and our pharmaceutical industry tell us their system is falling apart.

The type of administrative hassle that most rankles physicians involves not just paperwork but sometimes lengthy phone conversations required from managed-care organizations to obtain approval for patient referrals and/or diagnostic testing. Again, resources and time are diverted from patient care under the guise of controlling costs—costs that are then shifted to pay for administrative personnel. "Cost-shifting" used to mean using the receipts from private and government insurance to pay for indigent care. But our new definition of cost-shifting is taking resources from patient care to use for administration, profits, consultants, and, yes, paperwork.

Fraud and Abuse

THERE HAVE ALWAYS BEEN paperwork requirements in health care, and physicians have always complained about them: chart work, operative notes, transfer notes, and completing medical records in general. But the new brand of paperwork that has come about with managed care and anti-fraud efforts has added a whole new dimension, including new armies of bureaucratic personnel, to the paperwork nightmare.

In the private sector, the fragmentation of our system and the bureaucratic demands of managed care have driven the explosion of paperwork. A recent study of 2277 people in the Seattle health insurance market found that they were covered by 755 different health insurance policies and 189 different health care plans.[11] But for the government programs, Medicare and Medicaid, a different cause is driving the paperwork monster. That cause pretty much boils down to an attempt to control fraud and abuse. Many players in American health care, following the gods of the entrepreneurial spirit, became a bit too zealous in the way they were gaming the system. Some of the "abuse" was out-and-out criminal fraud, perpetuated by people outside the system. The latter group found it easy, especially with the opportunities presented by electronic billing, to rob big bucks. When HCFA admitted that it had paid out $23 billion too much through fraudulent or inflated Medicare billings in 1998, people seemed to blame Medicare. But it wasn't Medicare that did the billings. It was the providers or crooks who submitted the inflated or fraudulent charges.

HCA/Columbia, the nation's largest for-profit hospital chain, systematically overcoded diagnoses to bilk Medicare. This was but one of their questionable practices to maximize their billings. They paid a "first installment" fine of $740 million to Medicare as part of a settlement. Even Illinois Blue Cross paid a fine of $140 million for ripping off Medicare. Nursing homes and a large number of bandit or fly-by-night home health agencies figured out ways to maximize charges, even for services not delivered.

Mental health has proven to be a prime profit center (through fraud) for both corporations that have mental health facilities and individuals who run "shelter homes." Some psychiatric hospitals were keeping patients for just as long as their insurance paid the bill, with little regard for the need. Tenet paid a $300 million fine for that practice. A series of articles in *The New York Times* has highlighted the abusive practices in the group shelter homes that house many of the mentally ill in New York City. Greed appears to be the driving motivation in their care. Many of the patients were subjected to assembly line-type surgeries, like prostate resections and cataract repairs, often with questionable indications. The profit motivation may have led to collusion between the shelter homes and greedy surgeons, who were able to bill Medicare or Medicaid for the procedures whether they were needed or not. The federal programs have also been systematically overbilled by diagnostic laboratories, which paid fines in the hundreds of millions of dollars and then kept on operating.

In the field of "durable medical equipment," the situation is wild. I recently got a card from a supplier outlining exactly what I needed to provide in the form of paperwork so that a fully ambulatory patient could get a motorized wheelchair. There was no indication of cost, and I suspect it would have been close to $5000. The item, moreover, was unnecessary. The patient walked out of my office with relative ease. The markups on these items are incredible. Another one of my elderly patients, who had been hospitalized a few months earlier, had been discharged from the hospital with an oxygen concentrator for which Medicare was being billed $472 a month. At that price, she had assumed she was buying the machine (not so). She rarely used it. She informed me (I was totally unaware) that the renting company would not stop billing Medicare until I wrote an order to discontinue the machine.

Our system has also spawned a certain degree of patient fraud and abuse, though, dollar-wise, it is of a much lower order of magnitude compared to corporate stealing. The diversion and misuse of prescriptions, often related to substance abuse, has been a problem, especially with Medicaid. As a result, there has been a need for a growing bureaucracy to respond to the entrepreneurial efforts of some individuals.

Malcolm Sparrow, in his book, *License to Steal,*[12] goes into carefully documented detail to describe the extent to which fraud has undermined our American health care system. I get angry when I think of the care that my patients have effectively been denied because so much money has been diverted to what amounts to banditry, mostly of the corporate variety. The resultant mushrooming of administrative requirements adds insult to injury.

The Paperwork Could Get Worse

UNFORTUNATELY, THE PAPERWORK MONSTER could very easily get even worse in the near future. There are some experts who, in the belief that a single-payer government-directed solution is politically impossible, advocate for making the system *more* complex. They feel that it will take a greater degree of complexity to get more Americans insured. The types of solutions being suggested include vouchers, refundable tax credits, and employer-defined contributions. These all would (a) increase the already ridiculous level of complexity in our health care financing system (thus increasing administrative costs and inequities) and (b) make health care even more unaffordable for low-income people.

Part of the solution to our present and future administrative and paperwork mess could come from improved electronic information systems. They have the potential to make the health care system more efficient and accountable as opposed to creating opportunities for stealing. Computer networks, electronic medical records, and the Internet all have great promise as tools to help improve our system. They could be especially effective in the dissemination of information and in the improvement of quality.

In practice, however, the information age is barely beyond its infancy in its day-to-day application to the practice of medicine. I'm not sure the patient visit aspect of health care will ever become as fully electronic as the financial side has become. And probably it shouldn't, despite the efforts of Newt Gingrich and some corporations to digitalize medicine (e.g., the "Leapfrog Group") in the name of preventing errors.

Underutilization/Overutilization: (1) The "Underutilizers"

IT SEEMS ODD THAT knowledgeable people in the field of health care can argue over whether America's system suffers from too much underutilization or too much overutilization. There's no doubt that our schizophrenic health care system has both. And both have played an important role in the failure of our system to meet the needs of our nation. We have created a system with the wrong incentives.

In my practice I largely see a bias towards underutilization since nearly all of my patients are either uninsured or underinsured. Most of my Medicare patients qualify for the latter as they are predominantly low-income seniors who have a difficult time paying for their medications, even with our help. Ironically, our safety-net clinics now see a growing number of people who have insurance. They come to us because they can't afford their deductibles and co-pays—or when they have been turned away elsewhere because their insurance has too many exceptions or limiting conditions. One evening, I took care of a young woman who came to our clinic because she didn't have enough cash to pay for a visit elsewhere. Her plan required substantial co-payments for visits and full cash payment for prescriptions with reimbursement later. I had to be sure to prescribe inexpensive medications.

Because of the lack of insurance, as well as the barriers created by unaffordable deductibles and co-payments, people delay care until they're really sick. By and large, they have too much pride to ask for handouts from friends or family to cover the costs of care. So they often wait until they're *really* sick, like the 24-year-old woman who, fearful of the cost, waited several days to come to our clinic and then died the following day from a bacterial infection of her heart.

People with chronic diseases don't return for follow-up visits when they should. They ration their medicines, take a pill every other day when they're supposed to take it daily or just quit the medicines altogether "because they feel okay." They don't like being badgered for payment, even for the co-pays they can't afford, so they sometimes return a year or two later, when they can no longer get their medications refilled. Some may have run out of their drugs a few months earlier, and they come in with very high blood sugars or elevated blood pressures. When they have catastrophes, like a heart attack, a stroke, or sudden blindness from a bleed in their eye, they're more expensive to treat and, of course, their suffering is greater.

Underutilization by Medicare beneficiaries is a phenomenon I see on an almost daily basis. With the changing economics of health care, Medicare has become a form of *under*insurance. This metamorphosis has come about largely because of the lack of pharmaceutical coverage. When Medicare began in 1965, there were few expensive drugs. A study published in *JAMA* in 2000 by the RAND group on the utilization of services in Medicare fee-for-service (period 1994-1996) showed widespread underutilization of services deemed "necessary." This discrepancy was especially notable among black beneficiaries and in low-income areas. [13]

Underutilization is likely to become even more widespread in the near future as the cost of care rises and as employers increasingly shift more of the costs to employees. With a rising rate of unemployment, employers will feel less pressure to be generous with health care benefits. Employers are working with insurance companies to develop "defined-contribution" or "employee-driven" health care plans that give the appearance that they offer "more choice." But in fact, as with medical savings accounts, for low-income Americans, as opposed to high-income people, these plans will only increase inequities in our health care system. Low-income people will pick the least expensive plans with the highest deductibles and co-pays because that will be all they can afford. And they will delay needed care. They will underutilize.

The strategy to increase deductibles and co-pays is based on the theory that these higher payments will discourage unnecessary use of services. But insurers and employers can't possibly *not* realize that these increased costs will also discourage the use of *necessary* care, most notably for lower-income people who are truly sick.

In the more global picture, underutilization is a major reason, if not *the* major reason, for our country's poor performance on the major health indicators vis-à-vis the other developed countries.

Critics have blamed our poor performance on poor folks who don't comply with their care. Well, of course, those poor folks, especially those from minority ethnic groups, don't comply. The system wasn't designed for them and their chaotic lives. That's the major reason for the existence of our "safety-net" clinics: the community health centers, the county hospitals, and the "health care for the homeless" programs.

But when we admonish these people for not complying, we're blaming the victims. We've created a health care system that creates barriers to their access to care. It's low-income people who go without the care, who raise our infant mortality rate and lower our life expectancy rate. They underutilize mostly because they can't afford it. Their resulting poor health creates a vicious cycle of poverty, and, in the long run, affects our economic status—and our dignity—as a nation.

(2) The "Overutilizers"

THE CONTRASTING PHENOMENON, THE overutilization of health care services, drains our system's resources while providing minimal added benefit—or even leading to harm. Overutilization, or even "alleged" overutilizaton, real or not real, has pushed insurers to increase deductibles and co-pays. Although lofty expectations from consumers do have a role in causing our system to be so expensive, the insane pricing of American health care is much more to blame. In allowing prices to evolve in such an irrational and counterproductive manner (where quality and reason have been eclipsed by the entrepreneurial spirit), "the market" has done a disservice to America's health care system and to the millions of Americans who must beg for care or do without. Then add to the inflated pricing the health care industry's lavish advertising campaigns and the media's hype on new technologies, and we have a formula for the hyperutilization of expensive services.

What about "entitlement chutzpah," the rationale behind the alleged overutilization and abuse of the system carried out by people who show up at ungodly hours at the ER? The people who demand care for trivial problems because they have Medicaid, and that covers all the charges, so why should they care? So goes the refrain from the docs who complain. I suspect that the people (docs and others) who gripe about Medicaid "abusers" are somewhat less upset by the "abuses" of people who have private insurance or adequate cash in hand. Prejudice against Medicaid recipients has likely become worse as people with commercial insurance have found themselves increasingly affected by higher out-of-pocket expenses. The Medicaid package is much more comprehensive and consumer-friendly than private insurance, and, therefore, is often resented by people who must suffer high deductibles and co-pays. In Idaho, legislators cynically refer to Medicaid as "the gold card." The elements of class and racial discrimination also are a factor in the anti-entitlement sentiment so prevalent among many conservatives in America. The bias against minorities, even when they're insured, was documented in a recent study.

Yet, overutilization by poor people of color, or poor whites from Appalachia, with entitlements (Medicaid) constitutes only a minimal portion of the unnecessarily high spending of our health care system. All the evidence shows that poor people, even those with Medicaid, get fewer services, especially expensive services like cardiac catheterization, than middle-class people. The uninsured only use about 60 percent of the services used by the insured. It's more the high expectations of middle-class America, along with the willingness of providers to satisfy those expectations, that has led to the costly overutilization of expensive services. The word "expensive" is key. In Japan, with universal coverage and an average of 16 patient visits a year compared to about 6 in the U.S.,[14] they spend less than half of what we spend on health care despite the apparent gross overutilization.

Our American health care "monster" has created a situation where market hype has combined with (and helped create) inflated consumer expectations. The result has been a series of bizarre consequences, including inappropriate overutilization, as opposed to inappropriate underutilization by those who lack easy access. Unfortunately, as a result of perverse incentives, those least able to participate in the system have been penalized most. Not only do the patients come last in American health care today. They also are blamed for the system's shortcomings.

How our system has evolved to create a litany of perverse incentives is further elaborated in the next chapter.

Summary of Key Points

- The American health care system is a hodge-podge, a complex nightmare that wastes billions that could be spent on needed health care.

- The health care and insurance pricing system is incredibly "opaque" and encourages waste, fraud, and abuse.

- The administrative burden of American health care is wasteful and excessive. It diverts resources from patient care and has created mountains of paperwork for health care providers.

- Special interest groups of the medical-industrial complex have systematically taken advantage of the American people and of the complexity of the health care system to further their own financial gain.

- Insurance companies and health care providers often "blame the victims," the American people, for the system's shortcomings.

Chapter 3

Monster II:
Perverse Incentives
Lead to Bizarre Outcomes

Mimi, a 70-year-old patient of mine who has high blood pressure, diabetes, and arthritis, came to me for a routine follow-up visit. She had seen her dermatologist, who, upon learning she had arthritis, suggested she ask her family doctor (me) for Enbrel, a new medication for arthritis. Enbrel costs over $13,000 a year, and isn't appropriate for osteoarthritis, the type she has. However, because of high demand, there is a wait list for the medication, which is used for rheumatoid arthritis.

PART OF OUR PROBLEM with overutilization comes from the demand created by physicians themselves. We have a system of perverse incentives and illogical pricing. Procedures are reimbursed generously, much more so than in other countries. And third-party reimbursement removes financial responsibility from *both* the patient and the physician.

Many specialists are prone to advise the patient to have more, as opposed to fewer, tests or procedures. Ignoring the recommendations of such bodies as the U.S. Preventive Services Task Force, they will order more frequent screening tests on the premise that they are being more thorough. Specialty organizations tend to have more generous criteria for screening that falls within the purview of their own discipline.

As opposed to the fabled "wait lists" of other countries, in America patients may have procedures or surgeries done *too* quickly. I've had patients with what I considered relatively minor complaints of knee or hip pain wind up with joint replacements the next week, even before they had a chance to do physical therapy. The otherwise healthy mother of a colleague recently was to have a knee replacement. She had a routine preoperative chest X-ray with a "spot" on it. A $5000 PET scan ensued and the "spot" was interpreted as cancer. Lung surgery followed soon after, followed by a cascade of complications leading to her death. The pathology report showed no cancer. Then there are the hysterectomies, the tonsillectomies, a host of orthopedic procedures, and cesarean sections—many of which are not medically necessary. Maybe if we had longer "wait lists" in America, we could avoid some surgeries altogether.

There's "Gold in Them 'Thar' Patients"

AMERICAN MEDICINE HAS AN amazing array of expensive "routine" diagnostic procedures, such as colonoscopy, esophagogastro-duodenoscopy (looking into the stomach with a tube at $40-$80 for each of the 26 letters in the word), MRIs for back or neck pain, prostate biopsies, sleep studies, and echocardiograms. And each specialty has its own "armamentarium" of costly procedures, the "bread and butter" of each specialist. Sometimes patients offer especially bounteous opportunities. One such gold mine comes from people who have been cooking in the sun for years to provide a crop of removable skin lesions (at $200 each) for Sunbelt dermatologists. And every pregnant woman is a potential $1000 customer for an anesthesiologist who will place an epidural block to control her pain during labor.

Cesarean sections and epidural anesthesia during labor are two examples of a synergy between the patient and the physician that results in overutilization of expensive procedures. Patients create a demand for the procedures, even if they aren't medically necessary and may, in some circumstances, be more risky. Physicians are content to go along. After all, a cesarean section is much more convenient for the physician. It avoids being up at night as well as the stress that accompanies a long, difficult labor, and it's quicker and reimburses much more. It also removes much of the worry about malpractice should there be a problem with the baby. It would be much more appropriate to reimburse more for a difficult vaginal delivery than a cesarean section. Yet cesarean sections are reimbursed at about three times the rate of a vaginal delivery.

Epidurals are not always necessary, but patients have come to expect them. Our hospital in Nampa went for many years without anyone receiving an epidural. I think what happened was that (a) other hospitals in the area began to offer epidurals, and (b) the anesthesiologists at our hospital suddenly became willing to do them. Soon all our patients came to expect epidurals, and, even if they aren't expecting it, the nurses often convince them they need one. There's even a rush to get them done before a woman delivers! I'm not going to assert that women in labor don't need pain relief or that they categorically shouldn't have epidurals, but, given the experience of many years without the procedure, they should be used more selectively as their risk is not zero. And they can add $2000 to the cost of a delivery.

Diagnostic tests can be very expensive. Some of the expensive ones are controversial and/or questionably necessary. For example, there is disagreement among experts as to whether liver biopsies (at $3000) are needed for hepatitis C. And experts disagree whether it's important to follow viral counts (at $300 each) for people being treated for hepatitis C.

Unfortunately, American medicine has come to rely much more on diagnostic testing than on knowledge and cognitive thinking. It makes economic sense, since the diagnostic tests reimburse much better than cognitive efforts. I'm forced to take the cognitive approach in my everyday practice because most of my patients can't afford the tests. Ironically, by getting fewer diagnostic tests, in many cases the uninsured may be getting better care. The expensive tests often have incidental insignificant findings (now termed "incidentalomas"), which must then be tracked down and studied more, incurring increased expense and risk to the patient. Tests create their own spiral of costs and risk. I had an elderly woman with uncontrollable hypertension. A study to look at her renal arteries led to acute renal failure and a stroke, and she wound up in a nursing home. Another patient of mine, also an elderly woman, had an exam to look at her common bile duct and wound up getting pancreatitis with a full cascade of catastrophes. She spent the next 12 months in hospitals and nursing homes. In retrospect (hindsight is always easier than foresight), some patients might be better off if we had longer waiting lines for nonurgent procedures.

Relatively speaking, surgeries cost even more. And some of the newer medications, like Enbrel or Remicade for rheumatoid arthritis, can cost $13,000 to $20,000 a year.[1] New technologies have created new markets and new demands—and high prices. Emerging technologies of the future are likely to make the current "new" technologies look like bargains.

Creating the Demand: The Sky's the Limit

How REALISTIC IS IT for Americans to expect to benefit from all these new technologies? Would *not* being able to benefit from the new wonders be considered rationing? It's a dilemma. We have created a health care culture with a "sky's the limit" attitude. Corporate America and the medical profession have sold the philosophy of limitless progress to America. Employers and insurance companies have tried to put the brakes on the spending through impersonal cost-cutting approaches that have alienated the public, but no one has dealt with the "great expectations." Commercial interests, through such tactics as the direct-to-consumer ads, have only fueled the fire of rising health care costs, causing *de facto* overutilization.

I fear that we have only seen the tip of the iceberg in a geometric acceleration of these costs. As an example, what if every American with heart disease or at risk for heart disease acted upon the TV ads they saw touting Plavix (a blood thinner)? What if everyone currently on preventive doses of aspirin were switched to Plavix? For the nation as a whole, the extra cost could be 40 million at-risk people, times $111 a month for 30 Plavix pills, times 12 months a year, or over $50 billion a year just for that one drug. New research studies that come out nearly every week, like the comparison between Cozaar and atenolol for treating high blood pressure, show the advantages of newer (and much more expensive) treatments. The cost implications for the cholesterol-lowering "statin" drugs are similarly astronomical. But the "statins" appear (at least for the moment) to be a truly effective and life-saving therapy.

Meanwhile, we have strayed from the ethic of health care being a public good. Surgical procedures are patented. Inventions and new products that have a potential for improving people's health are now commercial properties. They are sold on "the market" to the highest bidders, even if many were conceived and developed with public funds. And the motivation to develop the new products comes from their profit potential rather than need. What has become of the healing ethic in health care?

The Ultimate Overutilization: "Boutique Medicine" for the Very Rich

IT'S ALMOST UNBELIEVABLE THAT, in a country where there are over 40 million people who have no health insurance and millions who go without care because they can't afford it, we now have "boutique medicine" for the very rich.

This new phenomenon reflects the growing gap between the rich and poor. "Concierge care," as documented in an August 2001 Associated Press article, now enables millionaires to have personal primary care doctors, available on short notice at any hour. No longer does the multimillionaire need to waste time pursuing the usual paths of our dysfunctional medical system. For a price, quoted as $1500 to $20,000 a year beyond the cost of the usual insurance, the busy executive or tycoon can have the at-the-ready presence of a primary care physician. And there's no time limit on the visit. For the physician, it can mean seeing one or two patients a day while earning more money.

The whole concept of a personal doctor for the very rich or privileged seems warped, an aberration of what a doctor is supposed to be about. When doctors' educations have been so heavily subsidized by public funding, is it ethical that they devote themselves to serving a handful of people who are willing to pay exorbitant fees for care? Speaking from the other side, don't the wealthy purchasers of these services have a right to spend their money on a product that saves their valuable time and gives them easy access to information and services they need? Yet something seems wrong when doctors themselves are treated as commodities, like a market widget, to be bought and sold.

Rich people, including kings, princes, and heads of state from around the world, have flocked to high-profile clinics in the U.S. to get their specialty care. And, in these days of cost-cutting managed care, their dollars have been welcomed with open arms. In some European countries with universal-coverage systems, like England and Ireland, people who want to avoid the waiting lines of the government-run systems buy private insurance and get quicker, though not necessarily better, care. Even in Canada, where there is a national commitment to equal access for services covered under the national health plan and an aversion to "jumping the queue," there is pressure from more conservative forces to privatize elements of the system and, thus, give the rich quicker access to specialist services. A few Canadians, though nowhere near the alleged "droves" in the myths,[2] do "jump the queue" and come to the U.S. for care.

The "concierge doctors" are perhaps one of the most outlandish developments that have occurred in our imminent transition to a multi-tiered health care system. They are the ultimate high-end expression of the American style of health care rationing. As the "haves" get even better access to care, the "have-nots" are finding their access to be increasingly more difficult. Even Medicare, which some conservatives seem committed to privatizing, is in imminent danger of going in this direction. The new "designer doctor" phenomenon is worrisome for several reasons. Among them:

- It reinforces the concept of health care as a commodity.

- It highlights the failure of our system to meet the genuine needs of people. As long as we do not have a working system, those who can afford it will find ways to "opt out" of the system.

- As mentioned above, it widens the gap between rich and poor, a gap that is a primary reason in itself for the

overall poor health status of Americans, compared to
people in other developed countries. The corollary of an
expensive system for the rich is, most likely, the underfunding of care for everyone else.

Opting Out: An American Privilege?

MANY AMERICANS FEEL THAT when and if we have basic health
care reform, people who can afford it should be able to opt out of
the system to get "extra" services. Part of this sentiment may
come from the fears of people who are satisfied with their current
insurance coverage and health care. They worry that a new
"national" system may dilute out their benefits. This fear is
one of the major stumbling blocks to health care reform. It
was the primary reason that the promoters of a single-payer
ballot initiative in Maryland changed their universal coverage
plan to a multi-payer approach.

Perhaps there is a fair and workable way for Americans to be
able to go "outside the system" in seeking their health care.
Nearly all the European countries have this kind of "safety
valve." And we do have a model of this kind of practice in
America in the realm of education. Everyone pays taxes for
schools, yet they have a choice to go to a private or parochial
school at their own added expense. Hopefully, if the U.S. chooses to take the path of national health insurance (as I believe we
should), the "plan" will be comprehensive enough and of high
enough quality that people will have no need to go outside the
system for necessary services. The upcoming reform of Britain's
National Health System (NHS) has provoked this very debate.
In Britain, to improve their system, they foresee an increase
in health care spending from about 7 percent of their GDP to
12.5 percent, with the goal of building a national consensus
"around making the NHS the best insurance policy in the world."[3]

Closely related to the concept of "opting out" is the principle
of "choice." The health care industry has given prominent
attention to this issue. We are told that Americans will demand
"choice" and that any solution must be "pluralistic"; i.e., not
single payer. The rhetoric gets vague because the touted "choice"

is not real choice (which would mean choice of; e.g., physicians and hospitals), but choice of "plan," which paradoxically really means less choice of the more important variables: the doctors and hospitals. All plans basically restrict choice and treatment options. Even the impending new trend towards "defined-contribution" plans is headed towards less choice. As health policy expert Rima Cohen stated,[4] "Don't be fooled by calls for more choice. I think all Americans want choice of their health care providers. I don't see individuals clamoring as much for their choice of health plans, their...choice of benefit packages."

The "concierge doctors" represent an extreme option for the very rich to opt out of the system. Ironically, the concept of the "concierge" primary care doctor did not originate in America. The Cubans have been doing it for decades. Their system assigns a family practice doctor to about 600 people, whom that doctor follows and gets to know intimately. The difference is that the orientation is towards comprehensive care for a *community*, with a public health focus, as opposed to providing "super service" for an individual or a particular family. Maybe we can learn about community medicine from Cuba.

Competition vs. Cooperation

AFTER GIVING A TALK about health care reform at the City Club in Boise, I was asked a question about the growing competitiveness between the city's two major hospitals. In efforts to gain market share, they were duplicating services by setting up new expensive specialty units, a trend that has since continued. Now they even have competing helicopter services. I ducked the question, but I shouldn't have. It later became clear to me what was wrong. These two warring hospitals were vying for "market share." In the 1990s, financial considerations (and, for some, survival) had risen to the highest priority, even for not-for-profit hospitals, which these two hospitals are. But instead of cooperating to meet the needs of the community in the most cost-efficient way, the two hospitals took the path of competition. They chose to spend millions of dollars on costly duplication of facilities and services as well as full-page ads to compete for market share.

A front-page article in *USA Today*[5] documents how hospitals all over America are spending millions on new high-tech facilities to do expensive (and profitable) procedures, especially cardiac surgery. This competitive "arms race" reflects a lack of overall health care planning, but it is consistent with the perverse economic incentives built into our current system. These incentives give financial rewards to subspecialty operative procedures. Meanwhile, general hospitals, where many uninsured and low-income people must seek access to care, will suffer as the specialty centers draw away the paying patients. If these public hospitals, with their ERs and trauma centers, are forced to close their doors (as may soon happen in Los Angeles) because their paying patients have been diverted to for-profit subspecialty entities, the whole community will suffer.

Competition has been hawked as a way to decrease costs. Even Clinton's failed health scheme was built on faith in "the market" and the unproven concept of "managed competition." I shudder with disbelief when I reflect back on the '90s and the mad scramble for "market share." Even at our local level, we had

Reprinted with special permission of King Features Syndicate

long meetings and debated for months about how to form PPOs, PHOs, HMOs, and a variety of other alphabet-soup constructs. All these schemes were aimed at preserving or expanding our "market share" of that new commodity, "covered lives." Could we have really hired consultants at $375 an hour (we did) to lead us through a maze of absurd legal constructs in which patients were reduced to mere widgets of production? Not to mention the role in the production line that physicians were being forced to assume by the managed care organizations. On the health care food chain, only patients ranked lower than physicians, while the managed care CEOs and the high-priced consultants were at the top.

Health planning has been a dirty word in America. With the demise of the old certificate of need programs, anyone desiring to open an MRI center (or other diagnostic enterprise) and sell their product on a competitive open market is free to do so. But this competitive milieu only raises overall costs because the products have to be aggressively marketed. And marketed they are, just like whole-body CAT scans or new pharmaceutical products, without regard for whether they add any value to medical care.

"The market" works in strange and illogical ways in health care. A surplus of medical subspecialists actually increases the cost of medical care, and a surfeit of new expensive technologies also increases overall costs. Instead of lowering costs through competition, the excess of doctors and technologies creates more demand. Ironically, America has many MRI machines that are so much in demand that they function almost all night long, yet there is no assurance that the MRIs ordered really improve care. And now we have PET scans at five times the price.

In health care, it makes so much more sense to make cooperation the norm. There could be standards for which diagnostic tests are appropriate and when they should be ordered. There could be improved cooperation among physicians and other health care providers instead of competition. Care could be integrated. Duplication of services could be minimized. The Kaiser model, with salaried physicians and integrated care where all the physicians communicate with one another, makes more sense. The specialist can often be less expensive than the generalist in the long run because the specialist will sometimes recognize better when an expensive test is *not* necessary. The key is cooperation. Sometimes, I have a sense that we doctors are not working together as a team with the patient's good as objective number one.

On the corporate level, competition has been pretty much of a failure for health care. The "big guys" seem to have come out on top. Like the game of "Survivor," the United Health Cares, the Wellpoints and the Aetnas seem to have held their ground while smaller corporations faded. The result: an oligopoly of health plans, with less choice for consumers (a.k.a. patients in the old days).

As for the big pharmaceutical companies, they have been playing games, such as paying a competitor not to produce a drug, that make a mockery of true competition (see Chapter 1, Myth #11). Cooperation? The most notorious "cooperation" in the drug business has been the kind that can run afoul of antitrust laws. In this brand of cooperation, drug companies conspire to keep prices high, as in the vitamin scandal, for which they paid a fine of almost a billion dollars. Why couldn't cooperation involve some kind of joint efforts to produce drugs that are really needed, not look-alike drugs, such as a tenth new ACE inhibitor to treat high blood pressure?

Prevention vs. Cure

AMERICANS ARE GREAT AT coming up with quick fixes. A free clinic to help the uninsured or a bake sale to finance an operation. But we've done poorly in our long-term efforts to build a health care system that is responsive to the needs of our people. We're number one in the world for health care spending, but we rank much lower in value obtained for the amount of money spent. As mentioned above, our health care system came in 37th overall in the 2000 World Health Organization rankings. A major reason for our disparate performance is our failure to pay attention to prevention and public health.

Instead of doing our best to prevent chronic illnesses, like heart disease and diabetes, we develop expensive technologies to alleviate the diseases once they occur. New hearts, new lungs, new livers, new kidneys, stents in arteries, wondrous feats of medicine and surgery. But we bitterly oppose such measures as higher tobacco taxes, seat belt laws, regulations to limit pollutants, meaningful health education, and gun control. Part of the opposition comes from the American worship of individual rights, but another large part comes from corporate lobbyists who are protecting the financial interests of their industries. Public health does not have the financial clout to fight back. Prevention is lucky to get a hundredth of the resources that go to curative medicine.

A study by Yale economist William D. Nordhaus on the economic contribution of health care suggested "the social productivity of health care spending might be many times that of other spending."[6] He was looking at the increase in life expectancy at birth in the first half of the 20th century, from 49 to 68 years. Nordhaus seemed to be suggesting that our investment in health care is not so wasteful in general economic terms. But what he fails to mention is that the great majority of the health gains in the past century came from public health measures—e.g., clean water and air, safe food, sanitation, safe working places, traffic safety, and better housing—instead of expensive medical interventions. The stent placers and joint inserters have certainly helped the quality of life for many older folks, but their overall effect on the health of the nation has been minuscule compared to what public health has accomplished.

Our health care monster, motivated by money, has given little more than lip service to prevention and public health. From the point of view of the private practitioner, who is charging hundreds or thousands of dollars each time he/she probes some orifice or removes some bit of flesh, public health is fairly irrelevant. A place to get kids' shots? Where you go if you have venereal disease or need birth control pills? Tasks with minor financial impact on the system.

Even the health maintenance organizations (HMOs), so named because they were supposed to promote prevention, have (with a few exceptions) given short shrift to prevention. They have mostly hawked prevention as an advertising tool. After all, for the HMOs, it makes little financial sense to invest in prevention when their patients, who probably will have changed insurance plans or jobs, are unlikely to be still enrolled in their plans after three years.

In our $1.5 trillion health care industry, little attention has been paid to such really sensible and constructive documents as *Healthy People 2010*, the U.S. Public Health Service's blueprint of health goals for America in 2010. This blueprint includes universal coverage as a goal as well as a host of accomplishments in prevention.

Our failure to resolve the problem of uninsurance in America reflects our lack of support for prevention. Because the uninsured lack access to primary care and delay their care, they develop more expensive maladies, which, if treated earlier (preventively) could have been managed for a fraction of the cost.

The Malpractice Conundrum

AMERICA IS UNIQUE AMONG the nations of the world in the prominence we have given to the issue of malpractice. Strangely enough, were we to have a more equitable system of health care that embraced universal coverage, the malpractice awards could be greatly diminished. There would be no price tag to argue over in the "medical costs" section of lawsuits. I doubt that we have more malpractice than other countries, but we do have a large amount of medical errors (that could be potential malpractice) that go unrecognized or unchallenged. Thousands of medical mistakes—wrong decisions—never come to light because people don't know any better or are not sufficiently empowered to challenge them in court. In these situations, the victims are usually obliged to pay for the mistakes of their aberrant caregivers. Call it fairness, American style.

After leveling off as an issue for several years, the issue of malpractice, at the beginning of the 21st century, is again becoming a major cost factor. It also affects how and where physicians practice medicine. Because of the sharp increase in the amount of malpractice awards—they now average $3.5 million compared to $1.1 million in 1994[7]—insurers have boosted their premiums. The rise in premiums has forced doctors in some states (such as West Virginia and Pennsylvania) to quit their practices. Whole geographic areas are left without adequate coverage for some specialties, such as obstetrics. Although there is great unevenness in its effects, the overall cost of malpractice to the system has been often overstated. Up to now, malpractice premiums have totaled less than one percent of all health care costs. "Defensive medicine" probably adds another two or three percent. But the fact that malpractice premiums are once again increasing is worrisome because care will become more expensive.

The solution probably lies in some form of no-fault malpractice insurance, except for egregious or malicious deviations. But "no-fault" would require some consensus that we are all in this society together, all at risk at some point.

The existence of the malpractice phenomenon isn't all bad. It has brought some accountability to the practice of medicine. However, its application has been uneven and often capricious, and more often than not it has been driven by opportunism and greed. As for liability and health plans, it is only just that if the plans make decisions affecting health care outcomes, they should be legally responsible and pay for their faulty judgment. Of course, the mere fact that we have a system that can argue over health "plan" liability and "patient protections" is a reflection of how far we have wandered off course on the issue of health.

Employer-Based Insurance: An Anomaly

AMERICA IS UNIQUE IN the developed world in the way in which employers control their employees' access to health insurance. Our system of employer-based health insurance came about as an economic construct of World War II, when wage controls limited the ability of employers to raise wages. As an alternative, they gave their workers health insurance. This arrangement has led to some perverse incentives. Although most employees, at least according to recent polls, seem comfortable with the system, they are generally unaware of what other arrangements could be feasible. They also are wary of change.

Health insurance has become an extension of wages and a tax-free boon for both the employer and the employee. In fact, the tax-free status of the health insurance benefit constitutes a federal bonus of about 10 percent of total health care costs or about $140 billion a year.

The incentives are twisted with employer-based insurance. The employer can use the insurance as a recruiting and retention tool in times of low unemployment. But if unemployment rises, there is less incentive for the employer to be generous with the insurance benefit. So, with the increasing costs of insurance, and with an economic downturn (as happened in 2001), employers can see an advantage to shifting more of the cost of insurance to employees. Employees usually accept their fate, or often they drop coverage for their dependents because they can no longer afford it. But in an extreme case, schoolteachers in Monmouth County, New Jersey, went to jail rather than accept the school district's plan to increase the employee share of the cost.

For employees, who have become accustomed to regarding health insurance through an employer as a "given," the arrangement creates even stranger incentives. People get locked into jobs, especially if a family member has a preexisting condition. They turn down opportunities that might enhance their careers or make them happier because they fear losing health insurance coverage. They endure difficult and sometimes humiliating situations.

Seeing the inequity in the system of employer-based insurance, where the interests of the employers and employees are often divergent, many organizations, such as the AMA and the American Academy of Family Physicians (AAFP), have advocated for the end of this illogical link. It is surprising that small business, which covers far fewer of its employees than big business, does not push to eliminate the connection. It puts small business at a recruiting disadvantage, while big business is able to reap the tax benefit. In a Microsoft website editorial, Joseph

Anthony argues for small business to support universal coverage.[8]

Divorcing health insurance from being a direct work "benefit"—really wages, but not generally perceived as such—would level the playing field for business, both domestically and internationally. Foreign corporations have their employees' health insurance paid for outside the corporation, so their lower production costs mean that their American counterparts are put at an economic disadvantage. On the average, almost $3000 of the cost of every vehicle manufactured in America is in the cost of health insurance, giving Volkswagen and Toyota an automatic competitive advantage. As Robert Kuttner asks in an article that appeared in *Business Week*,[9] "When will business at last wake up, break the odd link between employment and health coverage, and support universal health insurance?"

More Perverse Incentives
for Providers and Patients Alike

THE CASE OF MY patient who is experiencing "health care financing by subpoena" is almost as outlandish as going to jail over health insurance benefits:

> *Kevin is a 53-year-old man who was found to have a blockage of his lower colon when he was examined with a scope. Even barium would barely pass through the obstruction. The surgeon felt Kevin likely had colon cancer and needed surgery urgently, but Kevin hesitated. He is uninsured and has few resources. Seeking financial help, Kevin spent two months jumping through hoops to get our county to help pay for his surgery. They put a lien on his house. And they subpoenaed him to come to a hearing—contempt of court if he didn't show up—to decide on his case. Meanwhile, he's feeling better, has no bowel complaints, and is gaining weight. Maybe he won't need surgery. But he's had the privilege of experiencing health care financing by subpoena, just*

one of the ways we rob Americans of their dignity
because they are poor and sick.

As it has evolved, our nonsystem has created a plethora of perverse incentives. Health care providers and, even more tragically, people who have the misfortune to be sick have been especially affected.

Because of the lack of any overall planning, the staffing of our health care system is incredibly inefficient and unbalanced. We have an oversupply of specialists, all eager and willing to carry out the special expensive procedures they have been trained to do. And we have an undersupply of nurses and medical technicians, who, because they are in short supply in hospitals, limit the capacity of hospitals to serve patients. With increasing frequency, hospitals are being forced to close their doors to new patients or divert sick patients elsewhere because of inadequate staffing. Meanwhile, an oversupply of administrators and consultants has sprung up to manage a system which is increasingly out of control. And our system continues to have a severe geographic maldistribution of resources, largely because of perverse economic incentives. Providers in rural areas get reimbursed less than they would in urban areas for the same services, so why should someone move to a rural area, especially if he/she is leaving medical training with huge debts to pay off?

Because of their debts, physicians have much more of an incentive to become specialists to earn more money. I remember an ophthalmology professor at my medical school (Johns Hopkins) impressing us students as we watched him do cataract surgery. "That's $200 [it would be $900 to $2000 today] for 10 minutes' work," he remarked, "and I do three of these an hour." That was when the minimum wage was a dollar an hour. Fifteen years later, I was still charging only $9 for an office visit.

The discrepancy is even worse for patients, who must suffer not only the financial consequences but also the pain and the loss of dignity. Today, if a person with a limited income does not get her/his health insurance through an employer, the insurance will be virtually unaffordable. Should that person be sick or have a preexisting condition, the cost of the insurance, if he/she can even get insurance, will be prohibitive. Moreover, the insurance companies will force those people to face an incredibly complex set of conditions and restrictions designed to deny them the care they need. It's ironic and sad that the people who need the care most are the ones who are most penalized. They are priced out of the market.

Even if someone has an employer who provides health insurance, often the employee has to pay extra to cover a spouse or dependents. Many people find that coverage unaffordable. In the group policy at our clinic, the cost for covering a spouse and dependents is an extra $450 a month. If the take-home check is $1000 a month, it's obvious that buying the extra coverage is impossible. And the more health care that the members of the group use, the more the insurance company will charge everyone in that group. One person's expensive illness can lead to a huge increase in premiums for everyone in a group, as happened with our clinics' health insurance in 2002. It's a vicious cycle that forces people to become "health care beggars" or go without. It's better not to get sick.

The Mental Health Scam

THE SITUATION IS EVEN worse when health problems involve mental illness. One of my patients illustrates our system's failure:

> *Ronald is a 45-year-old man who works for a major corporation in our community. His employer provides health insurance, but that insurance does not cover mental illness. Although his earnings are adequate, he incurred a huge hospital bill when he was hospitalized for a major depression. He followed up at our "safety-net" clinic because he had to pay his hospital bill himself and then couldn't afford his expensive medications.*

Mental health in the U.S. not only carries a stigma but is burdened with a financial penalty as well. It's amazing how much resistance we have to giving mental health "parity" status with physical health. We'll pay full-fee for coronary artery bypasses or heart transplants, but insurers balk at covering depression or bipolar disorders. Is it the old "bootstraps" mentality or "personal responsibility" dogma that causes this disconnect? Or the feeling that we're personally responsible for our own mental health, whereas our failure to eat and exercise properly doesn't count against us? Remarkably, only a few years ago, the first "ER" for Idahoans with a mental health crisis was the jail.

I know we've been duped when some of my colleagues ask, "What are you going to do with mental health counselors who want to have their patients come back every day for treatment?" My reply is, of course: the same thing we should do with providers who want to do expensive sleep studies or treat heartburn with Nexium. We need to have scientifically based guidelines. But the line of questioning from my colleagues indicates that the "merchants of myth" have done their job well. Taking advantage of a public bias against mental illness, insurers have persisted in resisting parity for mental illness. They have convinced business to oppose parity by using the timeworn mantra that parity "would increase the costs of health insurance and lead to more uninsured." All the evidence, however, points to a minimal increase in costs, not to mention the inherent inequity in ascribing a less scientific basis to major mental illness than to coronary artery disease. And, if we look at the cost to society as a whole, I would suspect that the adequate treatment of mental illness and substance abuse problems in America would save our society billions of dollars. Likely there would be fewer school massacres, teen suicides, people "going postal," and drug and alcohol-related disasters. We might even see fewer anthrax-laced letters. Veteran TV commentator Mike Wallace (who has had a major problem with depression) eloquently expresses the dilemma in an op-ed piece, entitled "Mind and Body," that appeared in *The New York Times*.[10]

The real culprit here is money. The insurance companies are taking advantage of the situation to minimize their "medical losses." Just as they delay payment to physicians for as long as possible to retain capital for their own use, they are trying to delay the inclusion of mental health benefits for as long as possible. Meanwhile, even people who have insurance that covers mental illness or treatment for substance abuse find their coverage limits them to incredibly inadequate amounts of care, such as two or three weeks a year of inpatient therapy. I'd like to see an insurance company argue *for* mental health parity. Then I'd know they were putting the interests of Americans first.

The Patient Comes Last

ATTENTION TO THE NEEDS of the patient should come first, not last. Symbolically, however, America has come to place the interests of patients at the bottom of the list, whereas the "bottom line" has assumed a place at the top. Some health care gurus, like Paul Ellwood, whose name has been invoked as one of the promoters of the "managed-care revolution," are now advocating that America reverse course. Ellwood, in a speech calling for "HEROIC" changes, says, "The emphasis should be on the health component rather than financial incentives."[11] He doesn't go quite far enough. In fact, he partially misses the point by not placing the patient, or at least the "health of the patient," instead of the "health system" at the top of the list. His "R" portion of "HEROIC" seems to reinforce our health system's proclivity towards "blaming the victim"; i.e., the patient. He wants patients to "assume greater responsibility for their own health and for the cost of the health care that they require."[12]

Physicians have often been critical of patients "who abuse the system," as related in Chapter 2 (the "overutilizers"). There is certainly a level at which "personal responsibility" should play a role. But the cards are so stacked against the patients in our system (45 percent of personal bankruptcies in the U.S. are related to medical bills) that the mantra of "personal responsibility" is like asking a school of naive minnows to swim in a sea full of sharks. Instead of complaining about the misuse of ERs, our system should be adapting more to meet the needs of people seeking care.

As for the drinkers, smokers, and over-eaters, the solution goes beyond the health care system. It involves society as a whole. It behooves health care professionals to leave our safe little havens in the health system to venture out into the political and societal arena. That's where we should be advocating for the changes that can deal more globally with the issue of self-abusive habits. We need to remember that all of us exhibit some risky behaviors at one time or another. Should the downhill skier who hits a tree be required to pay her or his own medical bills?

Discrimination against people who are sick or who have chronic diseases is a much larger, and serious, issue. It's the cardinal rule of how the insurance game is played and of how the system games the sick: avoid risk. From the insurance companies' viewpoint, avoiding risk (people who are sick and, therefore, potentially more expensive) is the key to staying profitable. In our nation, 10 percent of the people account for 70 percent of health care costs. In dollar terms, the average annual health care expenses per person in this top 10 percent is over $22,000[13] compared to the average overall cost of $4637.[14] Any accountant can figure out that avoiding this high-risk group and insuring only people who are well is the goal. For people with a to-be-avoided preexisting condition, insurers either refuse to cover them or charge a fortune for coverage. I have a patient (a single woman in her fifties with generalized muscle weakness) who lost her job and is running out of COBRA coverage.[15] She got a quote of $1000 a month from a major insurer. Many people are afraid to use their health insurance because they fear their coverage will be canceled. Personal responsibility for patients? How about corporate responsibility, some obligation to the communities they serve, for the insurance companies?

In the debates about health care, little attention has been paid to the needs of the patient. Maybe this anomaly has come about because of the false perception that it isn't the patient who pays for the insurance. The assumption is that it's the employer who is purchasing the coverage and is, therefore, entitled to call the shots. The employee, whose health insurance is really part of his or her wage compensation, is getting short shrift. There are national arguments over the business practices of health plans, controlling costs for employers, or cutting back on the Medicaid spending of state governments. Relatively little public discussion goes into the issue of holding down costs for employees or patients. In fact, as alluded to above, the trend clearly seems to be to find innovative new ways to shift more costs to employees/patients. In the shadow of a market where the costs of health care and premiums are rising rapidly (an estimated 11 percent in 2001 and 15 percent in 2002), many employees/patients will likely be priced out of the market.

The Market vs. the Patient

DESPITE THE MORE GENERAL acceptance recently that "the market" does not fit health care in the same way in which it applies to other economic enterprises, the market rhetoric—now morphed to "empowering the patient" and "choice"—continues. Unfortunately, for many people of limited means, the kind of increased "choice" promoted in the new "defined-contribution" schemes may be the choice to forego needed health care.

The failure of the market in health care, with the demise of managed care as we knew it, came about largely because of its failure to recognize that people were not just widgets. When people (and physicians) finally caught on to how they were being abused by managed care, they rebelled. And "the market" in health care, at least as we knew it, collapsed. Or, perhaps more alarmingly, it may be in a state of metamorphosis. We seem to be on a path, with new euphemisms, that still leaves the patient at the bottom of the priority list.

The dilemma of organizing "patient power" to come up with a patient-friendly solution, versus an employer or corporate-friendly solution, is daunting. Conservative belief/rhetoric promotes corporate growth with the assumption that a prosperous corporate America will mean "more jobs," with improved worker status (the old "trickle-down" theory). Whenever I see the words "more jobs," I immediately translate the phrase into "more profits," just as I translate that other conservative mantra, "personal responsibility," into "everyone for himself." The patients/employees are behind the "rhetorical eight ball" in America. Any plea for equity, justice, or fairness in health care is countered by the cry of "socialized medicine."

How can we make sure that we meet the needs of the employee/patient? The AMA proposal for health care reform, which uses the rhetoric of "empowering patients," sounds positive. It does take an important step forward by doing away with the employer-based purchase of insurance. However, in the AMA model, the insurance industry, the pharmaceutical companies, the hospitals, and the doctors remain in control. The "monster" survives. Merely allowing more choice of plan or provider without changing the system still leaves people at the mercy of the medical-industrial complex.

Unless we deal with all aspects of our "monster," we will not succeed in meeting the needs of our people. Until we deal with the myths, put the pursuit of profit where it belongs (in "widget" industries, not health care), and place the interest of the patient first instead of last, we will not be able to fix our system and return dignity to health care. Meanwhile, we will experience an expansion of health care rationing, American style: delayed care.

Summary of Key Points

- Our employer-based health insurance system is outmoded, illogical, and needs to be replaced.

- Perverse incentives make our health care system a poor value for the amount we spend.

- Cooperation, not competition, will make health care affordable for all.

- Our nation has ignored prevention, thus creating a "time bomb" for the future.

- We need to put the patient first—not last—in the setting of priorities.

Chapter 4

Delayed Care:
Rationing American Style

Ralph is a 37-year-old man who has uncontrolled diabetes and no health insurance. He is unable to work more than a few days at a time because of chronic back problems. Although his mother, who is also a diabetic, has offered to pay for his diabetes medications and his clinic visits, he is too proud to accept the help. He only shows up at our clinic when he has an acute illness, an injury, or is in need of hospitalization.

"One reason people dismiss the problem of the uninsured is that they don't believe people are turned away. They're right. What happens is people delay getting care. And when they get it, they are more expensive to treat."[1]
— Drew Altman, President of the
Kaiser Family Foundation

LUKE, A 60-YEAR-OLD out-of-work computer programmer with diabetes, pulled a handful of change out of his pocket. "That's all I've got to last me the rest of the month, doc," he told me. "I ran out of glucose strips last week, and I can't afford to buy any more until I get my [disability] check next month." Luke was in the habit of delaying his care because he didn't always have the money and was too proud to ask for charity care, even at our health center, which has a "nominal" fee for visits. Two years ago he went a little too long without care for his diabetes and wound up having two toes amputated.

90

Gwen, a woman in her forties who works part-time at a "big-box" store, had a severe intestinal illness with a high fever. She came in after five days, and I asked why she had waited so long to seek care. "Because I still owed you six dollars," she replied. She came in after she got her meager paycheck for $37 that allowed her to pay off the first bill.

Defenders of our current health care system tout the myth that everyone in America, including the uninsured, has access to care through the emergency rooms (see Chapter 1, Myth #1), so there's no health care crisis (Myth #2). The uninsured are not hurting. Yet nearly every epidemiological study done on health care in America has shown that the uninsured have much higher morbidity and mortality than the insured.[2] The discrepancy, moreover, is not just related to social class or economic status. Put bluntly, the uninsured, even middle-class Americans, delay or avoid care because they literally cannot afford it. And, when they finally come in for care, they're sicker and more expensive to treat.

We have rationing of health care in America. Those Americans who worry about the rationing of care, if America should move towards a health care system like Canada's or Great Britain's, can relax. We already have it, American style. It's a simple formula. If you can afford the care, you can get it; if not, you can't. The American formula for rationing is particularly unfriendly to the uninsured. They even pay more for services than the insured, as described above (see Chapter 1, Myth #9). They are billed full fee for every service they consume. People with insurance, however, usually are billed at a discounted rate that was negotiated by their managed-care plans. However, even the insured are being increasingly priced out of the market, despite their insurance, because of the ever-growing size of deductibles and co-pays. And it looks like there will be more self-imposed rationing in the near future.

Higher out-of-pocket costs are all but a certainty as businesses move toward "defined contributions" or so-called "consumer-driven" health care. Even Medicaid patients may soon have to pay previously outlawed co-pays. States trying to control runaway Medicaid expenditures may soon be able to obtain waivers from the federal government to impose co-pays on beneficiaries—co-pays that in effect will ration care. The short-sightedness is frightful. The system is looking at short-term fiscal impact instead of considering the long-term effects. The lack of insurance or the imposition of higher co-pays only leads to delayed care. It's true that medical care is not really necessary for some self-limited conditions, such as colds, minor muscular strains, or "intestinal flu." But the delayed care for chronic conditions (e.g., diabetes, high blood pressure, asthma, or depression) costs the individual and society much more in the long run. The example of my patient Ralph, the 37-year-old diabetic, is illustrative. A recent study examining the factors related to poor outcomes in diabetics found that "lack of insurance was the most consistent correlate of inadequate care."[3] We all pay for the costs of catastrophes like kidney failure, heart attacks or strokes, either through cost-shifting (as with the uninsured) or premium increases (for the insured). Delayed care is costly for everyone.

The Mantra of "Personal Responsibility"

So WHY DOES OUR society tolerate financial barriers that lead to delayed care when it would be so much more cost-effective to design a system that encourages timely care, not to mention the adverse human effects? We have created an ethos, and many people actually believe it, that we don't value something we don't pay for. The corollary to this philosophy would be that the more we pay for something, the more we think it's worth. For the uninsured, they're simply priced out of the market and they won't seek care unless they're in dire straits.

The insured are now being sold the myth that somehow it's better that they have more responsibility to share in the cost of their care. The mantra of "personal responsibility" is being invoked to cover the failures of the system. It's as if paying more for your health care somehow builds character. Meanwhile, the costs to patients have increased so much that even the insured often must delay care for lack of affordability. What is their insurance for? Don't they realize that with insurance they are already paying in advance for their health care? It's not free. Even if their employers are picking up the entire cost of the insurance, and that's getting to be an almost nonexistent situation these days, those premiums are really part of their salaries. For the federal programs, we have all paid up front for the services received through taxes, taxes that we paid in advance. That's the meaning of insurance. But the insurers want us to pay extra so that we will hesitate to use the services, even when they're needed or prudent to use.

Low-income people must make economic choices, and paying for health care is one of those choices. Although some state legislators envisage the uninsured as choosing between buying a second snowmobile or health insurance, that example is ludicrous. The uninsured people I see are choosing between paying the rent, buying food, or paying for their lab tests and medicines. They often don't come in because they haven't got enough money to buy gasoline to get to the clinic. A recent op-ed column in *The New York Times* by Bob Herbert on hunger[4] alluded to "the elderly look[ing] wistfully at food on television—food they can't have because they spend their money on their medicine."

Some Terrible Consequences of Delayed Care

HERE ARE A FEW more examples of delayed care—and its consequences—in people we have seen at our community health center:

1) A 24-year-old uninsured single mother of two who is very ill with fevers and weakness, delays coming in for a few days because she is afraid of the bill. She dies the next day with a bacterial infection of her heart valves.

2) A 29-year-old uninsured married mother of two who skips prenatal care because she can't afford even our discounted fees. She comes to the hospital two weeks overdue with a dead 12-pound baby; she herself dies of a complication of pregnancy (amniotic fluid embolus) as she's about to get a cesarean section.

3) A 63-year-old man with heart disease and hypertension, who delays coming in for three months because he owes us $12. He runs out of medicine, goes into severe congestive heart failure, and needs to be hospitalized.

4) The 16-year-old uninsured son of a clinic employee (we don't pay for dependents' insurance) who injures his ankle while he's away at camp. Care is delayed, the ankle is broken, and more costly treatment is necessary.

5) A 54-year-old uninsured man with a severe lung problem who is to follow up with a specialist but gives up on the system because he is asked to pay a large sum up front before he is seen. He doesn't return until three months later after having lost 40 pounds. He then requires hospitalization and rehabilitative therapy for six months for what turned out to be pulmonary tuberculosis.

6) A man in his early sixties with diabetes who had been followed at another clinic until he lost his health insurance after an injury on his job. Although his ophthalmologist continued to see him and do five eye surgeries, he stopped getting medical care for his diabetes two years ago and ran out of his diabetes medications a year and a half ago. He came in with his diabetes way out of control (his blood sugars in the 300s) and kidney failure. He had worked his entire life until his accident two years ago.

I see delayed care and its short- and long-term negative (and costly) effects on a daily basis. It's sad from the viewpoint of both economic waste and human suffering. The results are not always as catastrophic as in the examples above. Often the conditions get better by themselves, without a medical intervention. Sometimes the delays are of a preventive nature, such as the 35-year-old mother who just had her fourth baby and is unable to afford a tubal ligation because she doesn't have the up-front payment. We expect to see her back soon with her fifth pregnancy.

But there are so many situations, especially with chronic diseases and neglected injuries, where the end result of delayed care is disastrous and/or very costly. There are also the people whom we don't even see, who suffer silently because they won't come in. Although people have an array of reasons for not seeking care, the financial barrier ranks highest in their decision to delay or omit care. These Americans can be compared to many poor people in third-world countries, who can't even imagine being able to get the care they need. As a 45-year-old single mother told me when she brought in her daughter, "I have to set my priorities. I'll pay for my children's care, but I can't afford to get the care I need. [She needed to see an orthopedist for surgery.] I've learned to live with the pain." And so have millions of other Americans who are forced to delay care because of our failing nonsystem of health care financing. We already have rationing of health care in America—and it's getting worse. The next chapter will describe some of the makeshift strategies used by America's "safety-net" providers to try to cope with a system that forces patients to delay care.

A postscript:

Ralph, the 37-year-old (he's now 38) uninsured diabetic referred to at the beginning of this chapter, came back to our clinic in November 2001. He had suddenly gone blind from diabetes—retinal bleeding. With the catastrophe, he immediately got attention from an ophthalmologist who did laser surgery on his eyes (cost of about $5000). Unfortunately, the surgery helped very little, if at all. A blood test drawn when he came in showed he was in severe kidney failure from his diabetes. His creatinine was 16.9, his creatinine clearance one milliliter per minute (both extremely abnormal). We had no trouble getting him hospitalized and evaluated by a kidney specialist. He is now getting dialysis and waiting for a kidney transplant. Since he needs dialysis, he will soon qualify for Medicare. Finally he gets his health insurance, though it still doesn't cover prescriptions.

Summary of Key Points

- Rationing of health care already exists in America in the form of delayed care.

- Delayed care leads to more illness, disability, and death as well as much higher costs in the long run.

Inhaling Medicated Air into the Lungs to Cure

CONSUMPTION,

AND ALL DISEASES OF THE

THROAT AND LUNGS,

FOR INFORMATION ENQUIRE AT THE

PULMONARY INSTITUTE,

323 West Fourth Street,

CINCINNATI, OHIO.

Persons at a distance desiring treatment can have it sent by mail or express to all parts of the United States or Canada. For terms and information respecting treatment, send or write for a circular. Address

DR. N. B. WOLFE,

P. O. Box 399.

Chapter 5

Jumping Hoops for the Uninsured: Caring for Patients at a Community Health Center

Imelda is a 36-year-old mother of two who is in the third trimester of her pregnancy when she starts to have heavy vaginal bleeding. Because she is afraid of the bill, she waits two hours in the hospital parking lot while she bleeds profusely with a placenta previa (a placenta that covers the internal opening of the cervix). She has a cesarean section and develops a blood clot in her leg after the surgery. She is sent home with a prescription for coumadin, a blood thinner used to prevent the blood clot from going to her lung (which can be fatal). She doesn't get the prescription filled because she can't afford it.

THE SEPTEMBER 2000 CONSUMER *Reports* lead article entitled "Second-Class Care"[1] outlines what happens to America's uninsured when they develop serious illnesses. It especially spotlighted our "safety-net" clinics, the Community and Migrant Health Centers, and the difficulties we have getting diagnostic tests and specialty care for the patients we see. Perhaps I should be offended at being accused of giving "second-class care," but I think the article was referring not so much to the quality of care delivered at our clinics, but to the type of care that the uninsured in America receive in general. Robert L. Ferrer gives an even more graphic and disturbing account of the plight of the uninsured at his county hospital walk-in clinic in Texas. He relates his story in an opinion piece, "Within the System of

97

No-System," that appeared in the *Journal of the American Medical Association*.[2] Our "safety-net" clinics are like putting a finger, or perhaps several fingers, in a dike (the American health care system) that has thousands of leaks. Conversely, our "safety nets" could be described as a hodgepodge of leaky buckets.

Caring for the uninsured is a mix of frustration and reward with good doses of hand-holding, puzzle-solving, critical scientific thinking, and penny-pinching. It requires being a real clinician, which means also being a friend and an advocate for each patient, not just a technician. A quick history and examination, followed by a brief explanation and a prescription handed to the patient, is not sufficient.

For the past 30 years, I have been working at a community health center (CHC) whose primary purpose is to meet the needs of the uninsured. We haven't solved all the problems, as with Imelda and the many others like her, but we've done a considerable amount. We've helped thousands of people whose contact with the health care system would otherwise be limited to showing up at ERs with a serious injury or illness.

Why They Don't Come In

PERHAPS THE GREATEST FRUSTRATION for a clinician caring for the uninsured is the lack of appropriate follow-up. Seeing an uncontrolled diabetic who comes in once every two years, and who ran out of medicines a year ago, is not satisfying health care. Why don't they come in? The answer would seem to be obvious, and it mostly is obvious: the lack of money. We do ask for a nominal fee (currently $10, though some other community health centers charge $20), and many patients cannot afford it. Some cannot afford even the $5 minimum fee we ask for a prescription. The fact that the prescription would cost $150 if they were to buy it at an outside pharmacy is irrelevant. I also have patients who don't want to return because they know they will need lab tests, and those will cost money. Many of the newer medications, such as Lipitor (to lower cholesterol) and Avandia (for diabetes) require periodic blood tests to monitor possible liver damage.

Often, patients will bargain with me not to do lab tests. "Doc, I can't afford them."

But for some the failure to return for follow-up care goes beyond the lack of money. The reasons can be complex, but are rooted in the culture of poverty, something difficult for us clinicians to understand. In my state of Idaho, there are legislators who equate poverty with irresponsibility: "Those poor people should be out there finding good jobs, saving their money, and buying health insurance—not wasting their money on tobacco and VCRs." Yet, how many of us clinicians, or legislators, for that matter, have had to live with dunning by collection agencies, having our phones disconnected for nonpayment, or being grilled by a medical receptionist about our lack of insurance coverage? Or, worse, worrying about how we were going to be able to buy food for our children or pay our rent so we won't be evicted?

The stories about low-income seniors choosing between medications and food are true. That's why some of my patients stretch out their diabetes and blood pressure medications, taking them only two or three times a week instead of daily. And they come in three months late for their follow-up visits with blood sugars over 300 and blood pressures of 160/110. Wanting to avoid the cost and/or inconvenience of a return appointment, they often call in hoping to get their prescriptions renewed when sometimes they haven't been seen for over a year. It's frustrating for us clinicians.

When I ask my patients why they didn't return when I asked them to come back (my note on the chart clearly reads that they were to come back in three months), their first response is usually that they were "feeling well." Probing a little more deeply, I find the financial consideration, "I didn't have the money," is nearly always a major consideration. But often it's more. It's sometimes a trade-off between work and health care. Either they can't get off work to come in, or being off work means lost wages or even fear of losing a job. Sometimes they don't come in because they're afraid we'll find something bad, and that might require more tests or X-rays that are likely to be even more costly.

Then there's the wait at the clinic, and the fear that they will not be treated well or asked for money they do not have.

Pride is important. Many patients have told me—some even break down in tears in front of me—that they are ashamed to come in because they have no money to pay. It's hard for them to face emotional collapse when someone asks them for payment. They'd rather do without the health care.

I saw a woman in her thirties who was getting her Depo-Provera shots (for birth control) at the local health department because they cost less there. She had missed her shot by three weeks and was running a risk of getting pregnant again. I asked her why she hadn't gone back in time for her shot. She explained that the health department accepted whatever she could afford as payment. There was no set fee. But her husband was out of work and they had huge medical bills, so she didn't have any money at all. She felt ashamed to get the shot if she couldn't contribute at least $10 to the cost of her care.

For many of the reasons elaborated above, people put up with whatever condition they have. They learn to live with the pain. And then there is the whole issue of transportation, which is much more difficult in a rural area. No money for gasoline, the car broke down, my stepson ran the car into a tree, the husband drives and uses the car to get to work. So they're not there for the appointment. They often either have no phone or have had their phone disconnected, so they don't reschedule and we can't reach them easily to remind them to come in.

The Medical Visit, Prescriptions and Tests: Games We Play

TRADITIONALLY, THE MOST FRUSTRATING obstacle for clinicians, and the most practical barrier for patients, has been obtaining needed medications. A medical visit does little good if, at the end of the visit, the patient gets a prescription he or she cannot fill. At our health center, we've managed to solve this problem the great majority of the time. Since we opened 30 years ago, we have included pharmacy services, and a pharmacist, as an integral part of our program. We have a formulary and can obtain many drugs at very reasonable prices. We even have an almost full-time person who coordinates all the paperwork to get expensive drugs for patients through indigent drug programs. Over 1000 of our patients get their drugs through these pharmaceutical company arrangements. Other "safety-net" clinics are not so fortunate. They often work with samples or vouchers which patients take to an outside pharmacy to get drugs. To their credit, though it's not clear that their efforts are totally voluntary, the pharmaceutical companies have been supplying many of their expensive drugs to low-income people who cannot afford them. Pfizer's "Sharing the Care" program is one such arrangement that applies specifically to CHCs, including our own.

America's community health centers serve only about 10 percent of America's uninsured, although they have recently begun to receive increased funding so that they can reach twice as many people in five years. For the other 90 percent of the uninsured, who currently do not know about or have access to a CHC, the situation can be much more difficult. Even for a middle-income person who is self-employed or working for a small business, and who has a preexisting condition that makes buying health insurance prohibitively expensive, it's difficult to afford medications. Filling prescriptions for three common drugs like Prilosec, Lipitor, and Norvasc would cost about $400 a month. The affordability of drugs is becoming an ever-increasing problem not just for the uninsured, but for the insured as well. Seniors (with Medicare) who come to our "safety-net" clinics face the same problems if we can't get them the drugs at a reduced price. Our cut-rate prices (and the indigent drug programs) only apply to low-income people. If someone earns over 100 or 200 percent of poverty (depending on the program), they're out of luck—no discount. Even for a person at 200 percent of poverty,[3] $400 a month out of pocket for drugs is a lot of money, and sometimes the drugs cost much more.

For physicians, one of the most frustrating aspects of practicing medicine is the so-called "noncompliant" patient, the patient who didn't follow instructions or take the prescribed medicine. With soaring deductibles and co-pays for visits and (especially) drugs, physicians outside the "safety net" will soon get a taste of what it feels like to practice medicine where patient compliance is a fickle hope, where the physician must ask routinely, "Can you afford this prescription?" Physicians will feel stronger about the need to overhaul how we finance health care when they see more of their patients fail to improve because they couldn't afford the prescribed tests or medications. Of course, since many patients are too proud to say that they didn't get the medications because they couldn't afford them, the physician may never know. I have a woman in her late fifties with breast cancer who went for over a year without her tamoxifen (for preventing a recurrence) while her cancer doctor (and I, as well) thought she was taking it.

Most "safety-net" clinics have arranged access to lab tests at a fairly reasonable cost. At our center, access to such tests is no problem, unless they're expensive tests, like a quantitative viral count for hepatitis C. But many patients are still wary of lab tests. They have a hard time affording even the minimal lab fees we tack on their bill. It's even more difficult for them to pay the bills that the outside labs send them directly. At our center, our patients have "in-house" access (at reduced fees) to basic X-rays and a few common procedures, such as colposcopy (an exam of the cervix) and obstetrical ultrasound. Other clinics are not always so lucky, and their uninsured patients must often fend for themselves in paying for these tests. As clinicians, we can order a test; e.g., a chest X-ray to be done at the hospital, but then the patient must come up with the cash to pay for it as well as the separate bill they'll get from the radiologists for reading the X-rays.

A Patchwork of Arrangements to Get Care

WHEN IT COMES TO diagnostic procedures, the situation gets much more difficult for both the clinician and the patient. Over the years, like other clinics, we've come up with a variety of piece-meal solutions that sometimes are wonderful for our patients but are often short-lived. An example is free eye exams for diabetics, but they need to be completed before the end of the month when that specific grant expires. These solutions have largely depended on a patchwork of grants, all of which require time and resources to apply for and administer. The paperwork is often lengthy and frustrating, but the patients do benefit.

The availability of mammograms is a prime example of the chaos that could be simplified if we had universal coverage in America instead of our current hodgepodge of financing. Up until about three years ago, only about 40 percent of our patients who needed screening mammograms actually got them. This number was undoubtedly less for the uninsured. "I don't need it, I feel well," they would say, or "I've heard they hurt," or they seemed too modest to have one. But then we got a grant from the Komen Foundation to cover mammograms for women between ages 40 and 49. And we got funding from the Women's Health Check program—with scads of intricate and frustrating administrative requirements—to cover mammograms for uninsured women between ages 50 and 64. Suddenly the same women who were saying "no" to mammograms were now saying "yes." Shame and fear of the loss of dignity create a host of excuses, which disappear when financial barriers are removed.

Our local hospital decided about four years ago that they needed to do more charity care. They offered to do free or discounted diagnostic tests (the hospital part of the billing only) for our center's low-income patients. Suddenly our patients could afford to get abdominal and pelvic ultrasounds, spine X-rays, even CAT scans. MRIs, however, were not included since they belonged to a different billing entity. With the free diagnostic tests, we have to warn our patients that they will get a separate full-price bill from the radiologists, but at least we're able to get tests that patients had refused to get in the past. Unfortunately, our situation is exceptional, and most community health centers (and their patients) must continue to contend with the same barriers to diagnostic testing that we had prior to this special arrangement.

Of course, our patients are still in a quandary if they need some other expensive testing, such as colonoscopy (an examination of the colon) or angiograms (injecting dye into the arteries of the heart to see if there's a blockage). Talk about "rationing" in other countries. We have rationing U.S. style, a step below the "wait-lists" of countries such as Canada and Great Britain. For non-emergency chronic conditions, many patients simply don't get the tests done until they qualify for Medicare (by waiting until they're 65) or Medicaid (which can be very difficult for an adult to do). Only if the condition is acute or life threatening will it get taken care of right away. Then the financial damage gets sorted out later, often through collection agencies.

Sometimes the condition isn't immediately life-threatening, but it seems sufficiently apparent that a test or a procedure is really important to be done in a timely manner. Then the caregiver and the patient, with the help of people like social workers, explore the options to secure financing. County indigent funding, service club grants (e.g., with eye surgery), applying for Medicaid, and asking—begging?—for charity care from the specialist are a few of the possibilities. So we play games, games that require a lot of time from a lot of people.

A case example:

> *Mary S. is a 64-year-old woman who was found to have "severe dysplasia"(almost cancer) on her Pap smear. She is referred to a gynecologist who recommends a hysterectomy. Because she is uninsured, she spends three months "jumping through hoops" to secure a promise from the county to pay for her surgery. She must pay back the county $30 a month "for the rest of her life," she calculates. Had she waited eight months longer, she would have qualified for Medicare, but by then she may have developed cervical cancer.*

"Begging, borrowing, and stealing" is what we must often do to get the needed care for our patients. Personal contact (e.g., between the referring clinician and the specialist) becomes the key link in the process. The referring clinicians develop relationships with individual specialists who are willing to help out and/or who have a social conscience. Unfortunately, there is often some negative fallout for these "good-guy" specialists (if they can be found, and, at least for us, they usually can, though it has become more difficult). They are often admonished by their business managers for not bringing in enough revenue, in contrast to their partners who are less willing to donate their services to indigent patients. And the "good guys" soon have their practices overwhelmed by non-paying patients, who are often difficult and time-consuming. Several of the "good guys" in our community have recently started to decline to see our uninsured or Medicaid patients.

Our hospital in Nampa is hurt financially by its willingness to serve our low-income patients. Since our physicians use and refer mostly to our local hospital (the other three hospitals in the area are too far away for our docs to provide efficient coverage), our hospital gets a disproportionate share of the charity care. The hospital radiologists (who bill separately from the hospital) have been hurt by having to serve our patients, who cannot afford to pay. As a result, the radiologists get paid less (the same could apply to other specialists), and the hospital has been losing radiologists to the other hospitals, where they get paid more. A vicious cycle. Or justice in health care, American style.

Why Do Our Patients Think
We Don't Have Universal Coverage?

IN AN ATTEMPT TO figure out why the uninsured are not rising up in protest to demand universal coverage, I carried out a mini-survey at my clinic. I did a very seat-of-the-pants variety of qualitative research using about 100 of the patients I saw in mid-2001. Selection was based on whether there was time enough to ask the survey question. I asked only one question, though I found I had to couch it in a certain way or it could be misinterpreted. Without attempting to influence their response, I posed the following situation: "All the other developed nations of the world, like the European countries, have made sure that everyone in their countries is covered by some kind of health insurance. The United States has not. Why do you think we haven't done it? Why are we different?"

Taking into account multiple responses, 33 percent of the people included "We can't afford it" and 20 percent said they didn't know why. The next highest reasons given, in order of frequency, were: "Doctors don't want it" (14 percent), "Government doesn't care" (12 percent), "Politics" (10 percent). There were some who "didn't trust the government" (9 percent) and faulted "greed" (also 9 percent). The specific targets of the "greed" respondents were the doctors, the insurance companies, the drug companies, and politicians. Strangely enough, an equal number (6 percent each) cited (a) the "fear of socialized medicine," and (b) the opinion that "we should have socialized medicine." A few of the more colorful responses:

- From a 70-year-old diabetic woman: "If they're doing it in other countries, we should do it here. We're the richest country."

- From a 48-year-old uninsured woman: "Too many doctors need to have a great big Mercedes."

- From a 67-year-old woman: "Too many hypocrites in the Senate that don't care. They think of themselves and not the poor guy who can't afford it."

- From a Hispanic woman in her fifties, formerly uninsured: "We let it go by. Before we were dumb. If you were sick, [you were told] 'stay home and rest and the next day get up and go to work.' "

- From a woman in her sixties: "The insurance companies have a good deal going. They do well from those who can pay, and not by those who can't."

- From a 52-year-old woman: "Insurance companies [are] the ruination of this country."

- From an 85-year-old man: "Health insurance should be like a standing army, protecting us physically."

- From a 62-year-old Hispanic woman who always brings me tamales: "We need to unite, get together and demand [universal coverage]."

Obviously, there is a lot of resentment, a strong feeling that the uninsured have been neglected and even taken advantage of. But many people, especially those who are the poorest, have accepted the fact that they're not insured. They've written it off as something unaffordable, and they aspire towards finding a job that includes insurance coverage. They haven't given the issue much thought. I have the feeling, however, that if asked, my patients could come up with some good ideas on how to remedy our system's shortcomings. They should be given the opportunity to have their voices heard.

The Positive Side of Working With the Uninsured

THERE ARE SOME REWARDING aspects of serving the uninsured. We have an incentive to avoid unnecessary tests and procedures. We must be cost-efficient in what we do because our resources—not to mention the resources of the patients—are limited. If we spend our limited budgets unwisely, we will be able to serve fewer people in need. That same motivation drives us to practice a more scientific brand of medicine. We also tend to stress prevention more, out of economic necessity as well as a perspective that (we hope) sees the larger picture. Our chronic disease "collaboratives," in which we have an organized approach to chronic disease, are examples of our efforts to join prevention with scientific outcome-based medicine.

We essentially work within a budget, and although cost is not our primary motivator (the well-being of the patient is), cost affects what we can do. Our diabetic patients don't have insulin pumps. They have a hard time affording the glucose testing strips that cost one or two dollars a day. But we do arrange free machines to test blood sugars, discounted medications, diabetic teaching, and (sometimes) scholarships for a diabetic training course. The "art" of medicine is important for us.

Uninsured patients don't expect to get every possible new test or procedure. They don't come in asking for an MRI for their back pain. They're willing to go with conservative therapeutic approaches first, so we see less iatrogenic (doctor-caused) disease. Also, we have many very grateful patients who appreciate the care we give them. Because we provide easier access to care, we're able to give better continuity of care, thus meeting more of the needs of our uninsured (or now, increasingly, underinsured) patients. Since we need to be more involved in their personal lives to be able to get them the care they need, many patients develop a more personal bond to the clinic and to our clinicians.

Outreach workers and case managers allow us to work "off-site" with the patients as well as add a more personal touch. Unfortunately, the relatively high turnover of our clinicians (at least in the past) has diminished some of the continuity. And the degree of chaos in our patients' (and their families') lives directly affects how our clinics function (sometimes also with a high degree of chaos). We are forever seeking creative solutions to meet the needs of our patients and our communities.

Community health centers have gone a long way to serving the "left-out" populations of the uninsured and (now) under-insured. But we're like a handful of fingers in a dike that is leaking badly through thousands of holes. In a recent study done by the Urban Institute, the authors found that, "No matter how the uninsured are supported—whether by third-party payers, the presence of community health centers...or local government subsidies—we find no evidence that these efforts have the ability to eliminate, or even narrow, barriers to access to the extent that insurance can."[4]

Our nation needs to wake up and give all our people an equal opportunity to enjoy good health with dignity. In serving the uninsured, we clinicians who do this work appreciate what universal coverage would do to resolve this "great indignity." So many (but not all, of course) of our frustrations—and even more importantly, our patients' frustrations—would be resolved if America, like all other developed countries, adopted a system of universal coverage, such as national health insurance or an improved and expanded Medicare for All. Instead, we are headed in the direction of shifting more of the costs to the patients in the form of increased deductibles and co-pays.

The next two chapters further explore America's worship of the mantra (myth?) of "personal responsibility," our growing trend to "squeeze the patient," and how many religious groups in America, invoking the same mantra, have (surprisingly) failed to support universal coverage in America.

Summary of Key Points

- The "safety net" has an essential role in providing access to care for millions of Americans but is an extremely "piecemeal" solution.

- "Safety-net" care is often more rational care.

- "Safety-net" patients are often resentful and cynical about the way our nonsystem functions.

- People who use the "safety net" would have greatly increased access to the care they need if we had universal coverage.

Chapter 6

Squeezing the Patient:
Co-Pays and Deductibles

Charlie Gomez is a 70-year-old man with high blood pressure and diabetes, both not well controlled because he fails to take his medicines correctly. Despite having Medicare, he does not come back for follow-up. He is ashamed that he owes us $52 and even more ashamed that he has no money for his co-payments. He winds up having a stroke for which he is briefly hospitalized. Luckily, it is not too severe but it affects his short-term memory.

THERE IS A STRONG feeling among many physicians and others in the business of American health care that everyone should personally share in the cost of their health care. Some even assert that people don't value what they don't pay for themselves. This philosophy ties in with the American creed of "personal responsibility," which is the philosophical antithesis of what conservatives term the "entitlement." Those with a more progressive or liberal bent talk in terms of human rights and justice instead of "entitlements," of health care being a human right, not a privilege. Language can define the parameters.

We're led to believe that rugged individualism—or is it really "everyone for himself"?—is the American way. And we hear much more about "personal responsibility" than we hear about our responsibilities as a society.

Idaho, the state where I live, is what could be termed a "bootstrap" state (as in, "pull yourselves up by your bootstraps"). A recent Idaho legislator suggested that the way a person could pay for health insurance would be "to go out and shoot an elk," sell the meat, and use the money to buy insurance. We could add this ingenious and original Idaho solution to the plethora of foundation-financed proposals for reducing the number of Americans without insurance.

Co-pays and deductibles perhaps in theory serve to reinforce the obligation to take an active role in one's own health care. This theory has major support from the insurance industry. But in fact the primary motivation behind the industry's support for co-pays and deductibles is financial:

a) Financial reason #1: If the co-pays are substantial enough (say, $20 for a prescription or several hundred dollars for the Medicare inpatient deductible), they force the patient to share directly in a major portion of the cost of their health care. The expense to the insurer is thus diminished.

b) Financial reason #2: Co-pays and deductibles act as a barrier to care and reduce utilization. The net result is a cost savings (at least in the short run) to the insurance company. In all cases, to a greater or lesser degree, depending on the financial status of the person involved—the deductibles and co-pays discourage or limit utilization. While this saves money for the insurance companies, it can be terrible for the patient, especially if that patient is low-income and sick. Co-pays, as we have seen at our community health center (see Chapters 4 and 5 above), often lead people to delay or completely forego needed care. Even for relatively well-to-do middle-class people, like many of the people I work with or myself, deductibles and co-pays are major incentives to delay care. How many of us have delayed preventive or other care because the financial disincentives have made us consider if the care was really necessary?

In an article that appeared in the *New England Journal of Medicine,* physician and economist Edie Rasell questioned the

whole rationale underlying co-pays and deductibles.[1] She
concluded that they failed to save money for the system. And
Canadian economist Robert Evans has noted that the effects of
individual cost-savings are illusory if they do not save money
for health care expenditures overall.[2] Indeed, the United States,
with the highest rates of co-pays and deductibles of any of the
developed countries, has by far the highest rate of spending for
health care.

Why Do Physicians Support Co-Pays?

MANY PHYSICIANS SUPPORT THE concept of co-pays as a tool to put
the brakes on overutilization. However, it's not totally clear to me
why physicians should be so concerned about what they consider
to be overutilization, or what benefit they personally derive from
limiting utilization in general. Are they lazy? Maybe they don't
want to be bothered by problems they consider trivial. Maybe
they don't like being awakened at 3 a.m. for those same trivial
problems. Possibly they resent a certain attitude they sense from
insured patients, especially from people with Medicaid, an attitude that seems to invoke the idea of "entitlement." I remember
one local doctor who seemed quite offended when I talked
about health care being a human right. "Does that mean that if
they come to me for care, I can't refuse to take care of them?" he
questioned angrily.

Some of the physicians' hard feelings about overutilization
undoubtedly do come from experience. Nearly every physician in
primary or emergency care has seen a Medicaid family where
mom has brought in a child with the sniffles and then asks if the
doctor can also examine the other two children because they too
have stuffy noses. Or there are the drunks who stagger into the
ER at 3 a.m. Somehow it doesn't seem right. The physician feels
that if there had been a co-pay, mom wouldn't have brought her
child in or asked to have the other children seen, or the drunk
would have thought twice about the hour he picked to be seen.
But is it fair to generalize from examples that seem to be "an
abuse" of the system and advocate that there should be co-pays
from everyone to discourage frivolous or unnecessary use? Of

course, the Medicaid mom or the drunk may not have considered their use of services "frivolous." And I personally regard many of these alleged "frivolous" visits as opportunities to promote prevention, such as checking on immunizations and healthy lifestyles.

In their first draft outlining their plan for universal coverage, the American Academy of Family Physicians (AAFP) recognized the negative effects of co-pays and deductibles in causing people to delay or forego needed care. In a break from the prevalent thinking in America about having the patient share costs, the AAFP in 2000 proposed a plan that offered universal coverage for primary care and preventive services without any co-pays or deductibles. They later modified the proposal to deliver only preventive and prenatal services without co-pays and to require a 20 percent co-pay on other primary care visits. They justified the change by invoking the "personal responsibility" paradigm that doctors and insurance companies are so fond of promoting. There is an inconsistency here, though it follows from the current conventional wisdom about payments for health care services. Are preventive services to be delivered without a co-payment because (a) they are so essential that the AAFP wants to be sure that people can afford them, or (b) the services are not valued enough by people who would forego them rather than come up with a co-pay?

As for the argument that people don't value services they get for free, perhaps preventive services and immunizations should require co-payments too. That way, people would value those services more, right? On the other hand, those of us who regard primary care as prevention, especially for chronic diseases, would argue that co-pays are inappropriate and counterproductive to good health.

Co-Pays That Hurt

THEN THERE ARE THE co-pays that even well-insured people have to contend with in the case of serious illness. I recently saw a Hispanic couple in my clinic who had a child with leukemia. They have health insurance coverage through his work, and their child is covered, but they cannot afford to pay the hefty 20 percent co-pay on their son's bills. What are their alternatives? Quit work so that their son can qualify for Medicaid or CHIP? Spend less on groceries for the family? Personal bankruptcy is a strong option for the insured family with a tiny premature baby that runs up a $200,000 bill in the neonatal intensive care unit if the family is responsible for 20 percent of the bill, or $40,000. Interestingly enough, the AAFP proposal deals with this issue by including a catastrophic insurance component in their plan.

The problem lies in the payment system, not in the people who allegedly "abuse the system." The co-pay protects both the insurer and the provider of services from overuse. But what protects the patient, especially these days when the co-pays and deductibles are almost geometrically increasing? We have a growing number of patients with insurance who use our community health center because they can't afford their deductibles or co-pays. Some insurance plans now even require their members to pay up front for all drugs, meaning that they go without when they don't have the $50 or $120 in their pockets to shell out for an expensive medication.

There's no doubt that there should be improved patient education to promote more appropriate use of medical services. However, that educative process should deal with *both* under-utilization and overutilization. Unfortunately, co-pays and deductibles, being indiscriminate in their effect on utilization, often discourage *appropriate* care as well as inappropriate care. They are often a significant barrier for those people who have limited economic means despite having insurance coverage. The uninsured, who are responsible for full payment, have an even larger economic disincentive to use medical services. Overutilization is hardly a problem with the uninsured. In fact, the uninsured utilize medical services much less than the insured, even in a "safety-net" setting like a community health center. Studies show they utilize services at 60 percent of the rate of the insured.

There is ample evidence in the medical literature about the negative effects of co-pays on the health of low-income families. From the RAND Corporation study in 1986 to a recent study in *JAMA* showing an increase in bad outcomes when co-pays were instituted for drugs in Quebec,[3] studies demonstrate that co-pays lead to decreased utilization of necessary care and increased morbidity. In the Quebec study, the institution of co-pays for drugs for the elderly led to a reduction in their use of essential drugs, an increase in serious adverse effects (hospitalization, long-term care admission or death), and a greater number of ER visits. I'm not aware of any scientific studies showing that co-pays lead to better health care outcomes, or evidence showing that higher co-pays lead to even better outcomes. Even in third world countries, co-pays have been shown to have a negative effect upon health status.

The failure to use health care services when they are appropriately necessary leads to delayed care, a frequent situation with those who are uninsured. And now, we are increasingly seeing delayed care with the *under*insured, or those with high deductibles and co-pays. Delayed care means more serious illness and disability in the long run and higher costs. It costs much more to care for a serious illness. In addition, there are the human implications of unnecessary suffering, disability and death.

The "Safety Net" and Co-Pays

IN COMMUNITY AND MIGRANT health centers, which largely serve people who "fall between the cracks" for financial or geographical reasons, co-pays or "nominal fees" are nearly universal. The exceptions are people with Medicaid and those who qualify for "Health Care for the Homeless" programs. The federal bureau that oversees these clinics encourages these fees, partly to ensure the survival of the clinics, but perhaps also to reinforce the "personal responsibility" ethos. Maybe one of our missions is to "build character." However, in my experience, the higher the co-pays, the wider the cracks become for people to fall through. Obviously, these fees help support, sometimes in a major way, the operating budgets of these clinics. To some extent they are necessary so that the clinics can continue giving the services provided. Yet it has been very difficult for our clinics to sort out which patients are harmed by the policy. Many patients fail to come back for follow-up or don't get the medicines prescribed because, despite the low fees of these clinics, these people cannot afford even minimal charges.

The Medicaid program generally has no co-pays. Where there are some minimal co-pays (such as for prescription drugs in a few states), they wind up costing more to administer than they produce in revenue. When the Medicaid program was established, the designers must have felt that poor people (for whom Medicaid was designed) did not have the resources to afford co-pays and deductibles. Although the lack of these payments is a sore point among many state legislators, it would be unrealistic to expect people with Medicaid to contribute any significant co-pay. Imposition of a co-pay would only lead to delayed or omitted care for the most vulnerable people, those who don't have the courage to challenge the system. People who have learned to manipulate the system will find ways to get around co-pays.

Nonetheless, there appears to be a movement in state legislatures to apply for waivers from the federal government (e.g., under the new Health Insurance Flexibility and Accountability Demonstration Initiative, or HIFA) so they can impose co-pays on Medicaid patients. They're looking for ways to spend less, but I wonder if some of the motivation for the co-pays comes from a desire somehow to "punish" Medicaid recipients. To put the issue into perspective, would we favor, for example, charging co-pays for the many thousands of New Yorkers who enrolled in "disaster-relief Medicaid" after the September 11 disaster?

The Larger Picture

THE DILEMMA OF THE co-pays and deductibles has two poles. At one pole there is the specter of a plethora of unnecessary visits by people who have frivolous complaints (the "worried well"), such as we're told happens in countries like Germany and Japan. At the other pole, we have the American health care system, where those who cannot afford health care delay or just don't get the necessary care. And there are even many middle-class Americans who *can* afford health care but delay or skip their care anyway because of the co-pays and deductibles—an economic choice which may or may not be wise. It's likely that the European and Japanese health systems may foster too much dependency on the part of patients, but in America, given the exorbitant cost of health care today, we may have gone too far in stressing *inde*pendence as the standard. We are systematically encouraging or forcing people to delay or avoid care.

Looking at the larger picture, (a) the overall health status of Americans and (b) the cost of health care in America, co-pays and deductibles, as well as the large number of people without insurance, are undoubtedly contributing to our poor performance on both measures as compared to other countries. Why do we rank so poorly—mostly 20th or worse—on such measures as immunization rates, infant mortality, and life expectancy? Do our financial barriers to access mean that Americans delay care enough so that they eventually require more expensive specialists and hospital care, leading to more expensive procedures and cost overall?

If there were no co-pays or deductibles, we likely would have a subgroup of beneficiaries who would overuse the system, just as some people do with Medicaid today. But, given our American ethos of personal independence and self-reliance, it's doubtful the phenomenon of overuse would become very widespread. Besides, the great majority of Americans, with a few exceptions, do not enjoy spending the day sitting in the waiting rooms of clinics or emergency rooms. Our American health care system has been perversely skewed by a philosophy to "keep the patients out," a philosophy which some medical residents pursued as if it were a badge of honor.

The transition of American health care toward for-profit HMOs, which benefit when patients don't come in for care, only served to reward the goal of "keeping the patients out." We need some balance. If we're committed to improving the "larger picture" referred to above (health status, total spending), and not just the "bottom line" of health care corporations, then at the very least we should do what we can to reduce the financial barriers to necessary care. And that means rethinking what we are doing with co-pays and deductibles. We also need to rethink how we deal with so-called "frivolous" complaints. Instead of creating financial barriers that discourage access to care we presume is "frivolous," we need to develop guidelines that can encourage care that is appropriate, cost-effective, and humane.

There used to be what was called "first dollar"[4] insurance, "in a distant land, long, long ago." How times have changed, at least for the non-Medicaid population. But what is the meaning of insurance after all? To insure against risks. What do co-pays and deductibles have to do with risk? The AAFP proposal places every American into one risk pool for primary care and prevention. Their plan is paid for through taxes, as opposed to insurance premiums, and it eliminates the co-pays and deductibles for certain—and in the original draft, *all*—primary care services. Conceptually, their original proposal could be looked at as having included (i.e., paid for up front or prepaid) the co-pays and deductibles as an *integral part* of the coverage package. The original plan did away with these payments at the time of service for the express reason of eliminating the financial barriers that lead people to delay or altogether skip primary care visits and preventive services.

I don't think it's a good idea, but I wouldn't be opposed to charging co-pays or deductibles for people who could afford them—if it were really necessary for the financial survival of the system. I think it's a good idea to have co-pays for expensive brand-name medicines when a generic or over-the-counter inexpensive equivalent will do the job. And I agree with a *full* pay requirement for services that are not medically necessary. But so often we have difficulty figuring out who can and who cannot afford the co-pays. And even poor people, like Mr. Gomez, have pride and a desire to keep their dignity. Must we continue to turn away the people like Mr. Gomez—with all the attendant consequences, like a stroke—because of a philosophy ("personal responsibility") that no longer has a basis in reality? In today's America, given the high degree of poverty, the difficulty in making a living wage, and our expensive chaotic health system, "personal responsibility" has limited usefulness for almost anybody, let alone a person with limited resources like Mr. Gomez.

Any one of us could be wiped out financially with a serious illness or accident. We are all at risk. For those of us who are caregivers, think how badly we feel when we take care of a person who has a personal disaster happen because of delayed care, a delay that frequently occurs because that person feels that she or he cannot afford the co-pay or minimal fee. It happens, and we all know it. In my own practice, it happens on a daily basis. As Harry and Louise speculated, "There must be a better way."

Summary of Key Points

- Co-pays and deductibles lead to an increase in delayed care or omitted care for everyone.

- Our high co-pays and deductibles likely contribute to our lower performance in key health status indicators compared to the other developed countries.

- Invoking "personal responsibility" to justify co-pays is a form of "blaming the victim."

- There is *no* scientific evidence to prove that higher co-pays lead to better health outcomes.

Chapter 7

Religion and Health Care Reform: "Personal Responsibility" vs. Caring for the Needy

God helps those who help themselves.
— 15th century French proverb, often
incorrectly attributed to the *Bible*

"It seems fair to me that in America those who can afford health care can get it, and those who can't afford it don't."
— An Idaho person who considers
himself religious

"How can any Christian read what the Bible *says about the poor and what Jesus says about the sick without hearing a divine call to demand that every person in this nation, starting with the poor, have access to health insurance?"*
— Ronald J. Sider[1]

MANY CONSERVATIVE AMERICANS, PARTICULARLY those who espouse more fundamentalist religious beliefs, equate health care reform with socialism, a concept they regard with disfavor. As such, certain Christian groups have generally opposed universal coverage solutions, such as national health insurance, that involve a larger role for government. More surprising to me has been the degree to which so many religious groups in America have avoided taking real action towards promoting universal coverage despite the obvious humanitarian need.

120

The struggle for health care for all seems so consistent with what religious groups are supposed to be about. However, beyond lip service to universal coverage in America, there has been little real action—with some notable exceptions—from America's faith community to bring justice and fairness to health care. The sporadic two-week missions to a developing country to "help the poor" are an inadequate substitute for helping our own health-deprived people here at home.

Part of the faith community's domestic inaction stems from being clueless. The way they look at health care in America has been influenced by the litany of myths propagated by the medical-industrial establishment. But much of the antipathy to health care reform from some segments of our religious community comes from adherence to the American credos of individualism and "personal responsibility."

Some religious groups, like those involved with community hospitals, have chosen to deal with the issues of the needy and the uninsured. The United Methodist Church has long included in its social principles the concept that health care is a right. A United Methodist minister, the Reverend Jackson Day, representing the National Council of Churches before a panel on universal coverage, declared that, "Reform of the health care system, especially to provide access to all, is not only a social, political, and economic imperative, but a moral imperative as well."[2]

Perhaps most notably, for centuries Catholic groups have had a strong tradition to help the poor and the sick. One of the most outspoken proponents for universal coverage in the U.S. was the late Cardinal Joseph Bernadin of Chicago. He asserted:

> *"Health care is an essential safeguard of human life and dignity, and there is an obligation for society to ensure that every person be able to realize this right."*

When a new effort, called "Covering the Uninsured," was launched in February 2002 by 13 major national organizations, it was the representative of the Catholic Health Association (CHA) of the U.S. who almost single-handedly stood up for truly universal coverage. The new alliance's stated major goal is to "reduce the number of uninsured," a far cry from universal coverage. Michael Collins, M.D., of the CHA, took a philosophical stand different from the (mostly) business interests of the alliance. He encouraged that "all Americans be afforded the justice [of getting]...health care coverage," and further stated "we cannot afford to leave anyone behind."[3]

How "the Market" Has Overridden Religion

WHEREAS "CHARITY CARE" HAS long been a part of the mission of health care entities founded or managed by religious groups, economic forces in the past two decades have often transformed the nature of this care. Many of these institutions have modified their formerly humanitarian goals so that they now appear to pay more attention to the pursuit of their bottom lines. With the evolution of American health care into a market-driven and competitive business entity, economic reality has profoundly changed how religion-based health care organizations, especially hospitals, operate. A result of this transformation has been a curtailment of the economic ability of hospitals and other health care providers to deliver "charity care."

Managed cost (*not* managed care), in the guise of "cutting the fat out of health care," took away their ability to shift costs to cover charity care. Indigent patients are suffering more, but in an atmosphere where health care has become an economic commodity, the concern for the poor seems to have shrunk to marginal importance. In a setting where profit—or, for some, financial survival—has become the goal, the indigent (who make poor profit centers anyway) have become casualties. It might lead one to think that the *real* religion of America is the pursuit of profit.

In this age of competition, as opposed to cooperation (see Chapter 3), many nominally "non-profit" religious institutions have evolved into businesses often indistinguishable from their for-profit counterparts. "No profit, no health care," has become an excuse to justify cuts in charity care. After all, they argue, if the organization (hospital) folds, there will be no place to give even limited charity care. Part of this change undoubtedly has come from their need to survive in the health care marketplace. But I'm afraid that the metamorphosis has occurred largely as a result of the transformation of the very soul of American health care. It used to be a calling steeped in caring and compassion, but it has become a market-based entity where business goals rank first. After all, health care now consumes one-seventh of the American economy. In the days of Marcus Welby, M.D. (the '60s), it was only one-twentieth. And by 2010, it may well be one-fifth. Does this transformation indicate that, in the American value system, the ethical values of religion now rank some degrees of importance below the values of "the market"?

Although it hasn't yet become an official religion, "the market" has become almost a faith-based value for some Americans. When I ran for public office in Idaho and campaigned door-to-door, I would often engage in discussions about health care, discussions in which seemingly educated people would argue for the market as the way to solve the problem of the uninsured. "It just hasn't been given a fair chance," they would say. The metamorphosis of faith in the market into the corporatization of health care seems to be a stretch, however, even for religious people who believe in the market. It's hard to justify the market as a religious value for health care. Market forces work well for selling appliances, automobiles, or fast food. But should we really be endorsing market values to determine who gets health care—in effect, who lives and who dies?

The Role of "Personal Responsibility"

Of course, it's more complicated. There is no monolithic "religious ethic" on the uninsured. Yet there is a very strong ethic, expressed mostly by conservative, but also some mainstream, religious elements in America, which clearly is in direct opposition to the concepts of universal coverage and national health insurance. This ethic colors how many Americans look at the issue of health care reform. It arises largely out of the oft-repeated mantra for "personal responsibility," the same mantra that keeps alive the demand for deductibles and/or co-pays.

America has been a society that prizes the individual, a society where the value of individualism has been given more importance than the value of community.

This "bootstrap" mentality colors our daily lives, but mostly affects those Americans with more limited economic means. It's a type of anti-welfare, some would even argue racist, sentiment that inconsistently doesn't seem to extend to corporations or agricultural enterprises that get handouts from the government. But it does discourage people who should be getting help from seeking aid from programs like Medicaid. It lends a stigma to being on welfare, using food stamps, or seeking needed health care without either dollars in hand or insurance to pay the bill. I've had low-income pregnant women refuse to seek help from Medicaid, even though they qualified, because they didn't want the stigma of "welfare."

In contrast to the mantra of "personal responsibility," the Reverend Jackson Day referred to a different kind of responsibility, our human responsibility to each other. He alludes to the story of the good Samaritan—poignantly, many U.S. hospitals bear the name—to illustrate the importance of social connection and "community responsibility."[4]

As opposed to looking at community needs, many conservative religious folks direct their largesse towards poor or excluded individuals or families. This approach is worthy, but it does not encompass what's really needed: a more comprehensive societal solution. But since that kind of effort smacks of government and "socialism" and could even lead to a new "entitlement" that might somehow diminish "personal responsibility," many religious groups are adverse to endorsing such a solution.

What the champions of the individual forget, as if they were stuck in a time warp, is that health care in America (as mentioned above) has evolved to way beyond the capabilities of "personal responsibility," at least when it comes to the issue of financing. Recent studies, including one done in Idaho as part of the 2001 State Health Planning Grant, have consistently shown that people below 200 percent of the federal poverty level have virtually no disposable income left to buy health insurance after paying for their "more essential" expenses. They can't even afford to buy the kind of "bare-bones" insurance that discourages primary care and prevention. Health care costs have grown so exponentially that even a minor illness can cost hundreds of dollars. Ask someone who's been to the emergency room with a bad cough and winds up with blood tests, X-rays, a diagnosis of bronchitis, and a bill for $500. A bill that must be paid out of pocket because (a) the deductible was $750, (b) the visit wasn't preapproved, or (c) they're one of America's 40 million uninsured. Now for a serious incident, say, chest pain, the bill could vary from a few to many thousands of dollars. The Good Old Days are gone. And so is the mantra of "personal responsibility" when it comes to the financing of health care.

Free Clinics and WWJD

RELIGIOUS GROUPS LOVE CHARITY care and "free clinics." Paradoxically enough, left-wing groups have also sponsored free clinics in America, with such names as "the People's Free Clinic," in response to the needs of people without the financial means to gain access to care. Strange bedfellows. Charity seems to go along with religion, though "justice" doesn't always seem to rank very high when it comes to access to health care. It's as if the more well-to-do folks who staff the "free clinics" can feel righteous because they're giving of their time and resources to "the poor." They become "good people" when they bestow their benevolence, on a very sporadic basis, to people in need. It's a similar situation with the religious groups of health professionals who give sporadic care—a week or two at a time—to people in a developing country with a warm climate. And these people sometimes seem to be more occupied with capturing souls than with delivering health care.

Religious groups are usually not as enthusiastic about community health centers as they are about free clinics, perhaps because the health centers are tainted with government funding. The real free clinics are often free-standing, sometimes informal storefront operations, where physicians (largely retired) can give a few hours a month of service time. It's a feel-good activity.

Because the physicians at these clinics usually have contacts with other health agencies in the community, the patients who go to the clinics often are able to access a variety of services. But often the clinics are an exercise in frustration. Piecing together a patchwork of drug samples to meet the temporary needs of the indigent does not make a coherent system. It's hard to imagine a network of tens of thousands of free clinics, manned by health professionals donating a few hours a month, as the religion-based "market" solution to the uninsured in America.

A few years ago, the Idaho legislature considered a bill that would make the doctors serving at free clinics immune from malpractice suits when they served the patients who came there. I initially opposed the bill because I felt there was a larger issue at hand: the legal rights of poor people. My preference was for the state to provide malpractice coverage for the doctors working at these clinics, much as the federal government does for clinicians who work at community health centers. It's a question of social justice. Why should poor people have lesser rights than people who can afford access to care? Individual compassion is great and wonderful, but it only goes so far in our current humungous world of health care. What the excluded need most is justice, doing what is right and just, so that they receive the health care they need in a timely manner and with dignity.

As mentioned above, my greatest disappointment is the failure of most religious groups to go beyond lip service for the cause of universal coverage. From the point of view of humanitarianism and compassion, it seems a natural match for religious groups to take up the cause of "Health Care for All" with enthusiasm and commitment. A commitment that goes beyond the minimalist free-clinic approach or the charity care of old. A commitment that reflects the complex and expensive reality of health care in America today. And a commitment that goes beyond giving a few crumbs to the Americans who are on the fringe of our health care nonsystem.

American religious groups should be an active force in helping America arrive at a real "systems" solution for health care that would provide the excluded with humanity, justice, and dignity in the health care they receive. As I sometimes ask religious groups when I speak to them, "WWJD[5] (What Would Jesus Do)?" I feel sure that Jesus would have been in favor of universal coverage. I doubt he would have opted for the piecemeal or "bare-bones" options that so many people in America are being forced to accept today.

MORALITY QUIZ:

ALLOWING 40+ MILLION PEOPLE TO GO WITHOUT DECENT ACCESS TO HEALTH CARE IN THE RICHEST COUNTRY IN THE WORLD IS (CHOOSE ONE):

☐ A) MORAL

☐ B) IMMORAL

© 2002 by Bob LeBow

Health Care as a Human Right in the U.S.?

THE MORAL ARGUMENTS FOR health care as a human right, as expressed above by Cardinal Joseph Bernadin, are not universally accepted in America today. Yet nearly every other country, including third-world countries, have such a right written into their constitutions. With regard to access to health care, Article 25 of the United Nations' 1948 Universal Declaration of Human Rights states:

> *(1) Everyone has the right to a standard of living adequate for the health and well-being of himself and his family, including food, clothing, housing and medical care and necessary social services, and the right to security in the event of unemployment, sickness, disability, widowhood, old age or other lack of livelihood in circumstances beyond his control.*

I believe that access to "decent" health care should be a "right" for every person in America. I feel it is a moral issue, and that is why I have put this topic in the "religion" section. Justice and fairness aside, I also feel it is to our nation's economic advantage to provide this kind of access to health care. A sick or disabled populace does not make a productive workforce. Even Thomas Jefferson recognized, "If we're going to have a successful democratic society, we have to have a well educated and a *healthy* [italics added] citizenry." The arguments about "health care as a human right" in America often get bogged down into definitions of what such a right would entail. Are we talking about comprehensive care? An "entitlement" or the "right" written into law? Health care on demand, including organ transplants and replacements of other body parts? The government paying for it? These are the kind of questions that we need to discuss as a nation, and decide upon as a society.

Cardinal Bernadin expresses the objective succinctly and well. "*Society* has the obligation to ensure that every person be able to realize [the right to health care]." Neither he nor the Universal Declaration of Human Rights state that the right to health care has to be provided by government or that the right includes every conceivable intervention. Practically speaking, however, there is a role for government in assuring that people have the right to a yet-to-be-defined degree of health care. And as a society, we have the responsibility to define that role. The process is called "community responsibility" as opposed to "personal responsibility," and we have a moral imperative to do our very best to bring justice and fairness to our health care system and to the American people.

"Of all the forms of inequality, injustice in health care is the most shocking and inhumane."
— Martin Luther King, Jr.

Summary of Key Points

- The faith community is inconsistent in its support for universal coverage.

- The market ethic and a commitment to individualism have undermined the seemingly obvious synergism that should exist between the religious community and the pursuit of Health Care for All.

- As a society, we have a moral imperative to define how we will ensure that every person in America has access to "decent" and timely health care.

DR. MILES'
RESTORATIVE,
NERVINE,
NEW HEART CURE,
Nerve and Liver Pills.

Dr. Miles' Medical Co.,
ELKHART, IND.

Return in 10 Days.

Chapter 8

Public Health:
We're All on This Planet Together

Juan Rivera is a 54-year-old uninsured farmworker who was hospitalized with fever, weight loss, and an abnormal chest X-ray. His skin test and other tests are negative for tuberculosis, and he recovers enough to be discharged from the hospital. He was to follow up with a lung specialist for further evaluation, but when he gets to the specialist's office, he is asked for $100 up front before he can be seen. Discouraged with the system, he gives up and decides to forego medical care. He shows up at our clinic several months later having lost another 40 pounds. His sputum smear now shows sheets of acid-fast bacilli (tuberculosis).

FOR THE SHORTSIGHTED WHO put faith in the mantra of "personal responsibility," there is a failure to realize that, when it comes to the spread of infectious diseases, lack of access to care can lead to public health catastrophes. In reality, we're all on this planet together.

Fortunately, Juan Rivera's tuberculosis turned out not to be a multiple-drug-resistant strain, but he did manage to infect at least one other person in his household, and perhaps others. Maybe our clinic could have done more to follow up on Juan, to make sure that he came back for care. We could have helped lead him through a maze of paperwork and bureaucracy that might have qualified him for some kind of medical assistance. In fact, because of people like Juan, we have applied for (and recently received) grant funds to hire an extra social worker. That's what we need to help solve access-to-care dilemmas for all the Juans

130

who need similar help in negotiating America's hodgepodge of a health care system.

In the past, when there were infectious disease problems, public health departments—at least where I was working—used to have adequate enough staffing to do epidemiological work-ups. They could both investigate contacts and follow up on people who fell between the cracks. Not so any more. Budget and staffing cuts have severely restricted public health capabilities in America.[1] Of course, in Juan's case, we didn't even know at first that he had tuberculosis, and maybe he didn't have the disease when he first came in. It's often an elusive illness to diagnose. But his lack of the means to pay for care—and his frustration and shame at being drubbed by the system—led him to give up even trying to gain access to care.

America has thousands of Juan Riveras, thousands of people who are on the street spreading their diseases to other people. Some of them are recent immigrants who have unrecognized and untreated infectious diseases. They may have multiple-drug-resistant tuberculosis, like the California schoolgirl who infected several of her classmates. Or they may have HIV/AIDS, hepatitis, chlamydia, syphilis, or infectious skin diseases. They may be avoiding care because they are afraid of what they might have, but more often they avoid or delay care because they can't afford it.

The paradoxical and ironic twist to this dilemma is that we all pay for the care in the long run. As Juan's case illustrates, once these people have a catastrophic event and gain entry to our system, they get the specialty care and the expensive diagnostic tests they need. Unfortunately, their care is often much more expensive because they delayed the care in the first place or had problems gaining timely access to our system. Juan wound up spending about six months at a rehabilitation hospital and eventually recovered—and somebody paid the bills. I suspect it would have been more cost-effective (and humanitarian and decent) to have made sure that Juan had received more timely care. Beyond Juan's personal suffering, one also has to consider the public health implications.

Public Health and Chronic Disease

TIMELY CARE HAS A public health impact beyond infectious diseases. In the area of chronic disease, such as diabetes and hypertension, delayed care has many adverse effects with public health implications; e.g.:

- A higher rate of complications.

- Increased mortality and morbidity (as from heart attacks, strokes, limb amputations, blindness, kidney failure).

- Increased overall costs.

- More disability.
- A greatly increased level of human suffering.

The inadequate treatment of chronic disease takes an over-whelming psychological and financial toll upon families. The cost to society as a whole—in effect, the public health costs—are also huge. On an individual basis, consider the financial, and human, implications of a 60-year-old previously healthy man who has a dehabilitating stroke that might have been prevented with adequate care. Perhaps this man's misfortune helps a whole industry devoted to home care, rehabilitation, and durable medical equipment. But the human costs for this heretofore active, productive person—and the wife who must now cut back on her active life to care for him—are daunting, to say the least. Multiply this type of situation by a few million and we have a public health problem of the highest magnitude as well as a problem with significant impact upon our nation's economy.

America has recognized the public health importance of treating certain conditions. We have taken a patchwork (or categorical), as opposed to comprehensive, approach to address some specific problems; e.g., HIV/AIDS coverage through Ryan White funds, prenatal care through expansion of Medicaid income criteria, or family planning through Title X funding. There used to be more local health department involvement in infectious diseases, such as follow-up for tuberculosis and venereal diseases, but resources have been stretched to a point where these activities are often impossible to carry out.

Access to care in a more comprehensive sense has public health implications. As such, there has been some recognition of the merits of population-based approaches to providing access to care. The recent State Children's Health Insurance Program (CHIP), enacted in 1997, has provided expansion of health insurance coverage for children (and, in some states, to parents) though there are still almost nine million children in America without health insurance. Years ago, we recognized that low-income people and seniors needed help getting health care. As a result, we implemented or supported Medicaid, Medicare, and a variety of "safety nets" such as Community and Migrant Health Centers and public hospitals. All of these approaches, for one reason or another, are either incomplete or inadequate. And these "solutions" have created a system that is at once unwieldy, overly complicated, duplicative, expensive and grossly inequitable.

The New Twist to Wake Us Up: Bioterrorism

Now WE HAVE A new twist with a public health dimension which further brings into question the validity of the old mantra about "personal responsibility": bioterrorism. Should Americans be expected to fend for themselves when they come down with—or think they may have—anthrax, enteric diseases from a poisoned water supply, neurological damage from poison gas, or even worse, smallpox? Will each person so affected be expected to show her/his health insurance card at the front desk and/or be expected to foot the bill, no matter what? "Sorry, you've got a $2000 deductible, and you'll have to come up with $100 up front before the doctor will see you with that blistering rash covering your whole body."

I suspect that, using typical American ingenuity, we will come up with a special fund, perhaps the "Anthrax, Bioterrorism, and Chemical Disabilities (ABCD)" Fund. The fund will have, of course, appropriately complicated screening and eligibility criteria. And it will pay for services related to the War on

Terrorism—assuming that other insurances are billed first, of course.

The whole emerging issue of the health effects of bioterrorism does bring into focus the craziness of our current system for financing health care. We are forced to look at how we are all in this together. We are a community, a society, and what some of us do affects everyone else. Terrorist retaliation for what we as a nation might do in Afghanistan, Palestine, Iraq, or anywhere else in the world can cause death and disability for those Americans who are unfortunate enough, like the people in the World Trade Center, to be in the wrong place at the wrong time. Obviously, the same dependence on chance and luck applies to accidents.

And a similar situation applies to a great degree, though not totally, to chronic diseases. Many of these ailments are more than likely to be caused, at least somewhat, by environmental factors and/or our genetic inheritance. It makes no sense, either financial or humanitarian, to continue our current way of covering health care in America. Our system is looking increasingly like a combination of two TV shows: "Wheel of Fortune" and "Survivor." Don't get sick. And you'd better not be sipping your espresso at a café when a suicide bomber walks in and lights his or her match.

In the past two decades, as the emphasis in health care in America has shifted away from "care" and the patient to "cost" and business, the role of public health has diminished. In implementing a steady rise in our co-pays and deductibles, the system has ignored the public health consequences of delayed care, most notably for infectious diseases and chronic illnesses. With respect to chronic diseases, the victims have largely been people of limited means. In contrast, the infectious disease threat (e.g., as with anthrax, Lyme disease, or multiple-drug-resistant tuberculosis) does not select out any particular economic class. In trying to discourage so-called "overutilization" (see Chapter 2, "the Monster We Have Created"), we have encouraged an ambiance of underutilization, a much more serious problem with serious public health consequences.

Public health deals with population groups, but it also deals with each individual. Sometimes the two objects of public health efforts appear to come into conflict, such as when WHO policy dictated when people should *not* be treated for tuberculosis—for fear of creating drug resistance and untreatable disease. And the same international debate is beginning for HIV/AIDS. The situation in the third world is, of course, different from ours. But, if America had universal coverage, our own "third-world" population would be largely freed from the ethical dilemma of defining public vs. individual needs.

Meanwhile, we're all at risk as long as we perpetuate a system that seems to be designed to ignore public health considerations, factors that have been assumed (incorrectly) to be of minor financial importance and not a positive force for the short-term bottom line. It's as if some of us (maybe the CEOs and executives of the insurance companies) are not on this world with the rest of us. Maybe when we accept the premise that "we're all on this planet together," and that—rich or poor, whites or people of color—we're all susceptible to the same public health (and other health) risks, we'll understand better why our health care system needs fundamental change.

In the U.S., we do have a successful example, at least from the perspective of the patient, of a systems approach to health care coverage that places some of us (those 65 and over) "on the same planet" with regard to health care. It uses a "one risk pool" mechanism, and it's called Medicare. Unfortunately, it's under attack despite its popularity among our seniors.

Summary of Key Points

- Everyone in America has a shared risk for infectious disease, terrorist attacks, and (to some degree) chronic illnesses.

- From a public health viewpoint, it is only just that the whole community share the financial risk associated with these events or conditions.

Chapter 9

Blaming the Victim:
A Bad Rap for Medicare

*"Whatever the solution is, we don't want more
government. Anything but big government."*
— A small business owner in Idaho

*"I don't want the government messing with my
Medicare."*
— An elderly Florida man, 1994

IN THE AMERICAN WEST, where many people—health
care providers and patients alike—have an almost innate distrust
of government, it is difficult to sell the concept of Medicare for
All. Physicians are especially wary and incredulous, especially
since Medicare began to crack down on billing irregularities in
a manner that doctors perceived to be arbitrary and heavy-hand-
ed. When Medicare cut its reimbursement to doctors by 5.4 percent at the beginning of 2002, all because of a flawed
formula based on the GDP, physicians became even more dissatisfied. Hospital administrators have also been extremely
frustrated with Medicare's onerous regulations as well as alleged
underpayments. As for the beneficiaries, although they are often
confused by the workings of Medicare, they appreciate the "safety net" that the program provides for them, even if it is incomplete. And seniors fiercely defend "their Medicare."

When asked how much overhead Medicare has, it's amazing
how providers and patients alike come up with grossly inflated
estimates. A gynecologist colleague of mine guessed, "It must be
70 percent." And I've had seniors in a polled audience figure

that it had to be at least 50 percent. They assume that since the federal government runs Medicare, it has to be wasteful. They believe the myth that the private sector is always better, more efficient, than the government. Never mind that 97 to 98 cents of every Medicare dollar goes out in payments to health care providers, compared to an average of about 85 cents in the private sector (see Chapter 1, Myth #4, for more discussion).

Part of Medicare's efficiency comes from its sheer size, an advantage that would be replicable if we had national health insurance. Other factors also contribute to its low overhead, such as: no profit motive, no middlemen or commissions, no onerous eligibility requirements, simplified forms, and no need to market a product. On the other hand, many providers, especially hospitals, complain that the regulatory burden of Medicare raises their administrative costs.

However, in the past two decades, Medicare has not been alone in causing added administrative headaches for providers. Especially for physicians, but also for hospitals and other types of providers, Medicare's rules and restraints have often been a lesser evil than the dictates of the managed-care industry. Even with regard to reimbursement, despite the complaints about Medicare, managed-care plans have often paid providers even less.

The Medicare model offers great opportunities for savings in administrative costs. As mentioned above, overall administrative costs in the United States consume an estimated 25–30 percent of health care spending. Canada's single-payer system spends less than half that percentage on administrative costs. If we could cut our administrative costs in half in America, we could save about $200 billion a year (based on 2002 spending), money which could be spent on patient care and prevention instead of marketing, duplication of services, paperwork, profits, commissions, and astronomical CEO salaries. These administrative savings alone could easily allow us to afford universal coverage in America.

Yet there is distrust of the government, a gut feeling—though unsubstantiated by hard figures—that the government (Medicare and Medicaid) is less efficient than the private sector.

Medicare as the Victim

FROM THE PATIENT (OR CONSUMER) point of view, Medicare's short-coming is that it's an incomplete program, not comprehensive enough. In a feature article on Medicare reform that appeared in *The New York Times* in the summer of 2000,[1] the Baltimore seniors who were interviewed agreed upon a simple message. They didn't want Medicare "reformed" or privatized. "Improve and expand it," they advised. But it's a different story from the provider side, which all too often feels put out and irritated by Medicare. It didn't used to be that way. In the "good old days" when Medicare started, over the objections of the AMA, it simply paid the bills that were submitted. What a deal. Of course, the "blank check" days had to end. Too many providers—and others who were just out to defraud the system without even providing a service—learned how to bill Medicare so as to maximize their income (see Chapter 2).

Even after Medicare began to put some restraints on the system, such as Diagnosis Related Groups (DRGs), providers figured out how to maximize their reimbursement by such practices as "unbundling" or "up-coding." America's largest for-profit hospital chain, HCA/Columbia, paid a first installment $745 million dollar fine in 2001 for the fraudulent billing of Medicare, largely related to "up-coding," or coding illnesses at a higher rate of severity than merited. Medicare (and Medicaid too) were being, and continue to be, ripped off, and then blamed for being too bureaucratic.

Congress became aware of some of the abuses and attempted to put more controls on the health care industry in the Balanced Budget Amendment of 1997. Unfortunately, their action did "throw some of the babies out with the bath water." America's "free-enterprise" ethic combined with the entrepreneurial spirit of medical providers may have contributed to the problem. Adding to the dilemma were others who were out-and-out crooks doing blatant fraud. Some of the worst abuses came from home health agencies, nursing homes, so-called "Medicaid mills," and for-profit hospitals. But the billing abuse has been more generalized. My former nurse, checking over the bill that was sent to

Medicare by the Pennsylvania hospital where she had had a pacemaker implanted, noted that Medicare had been billed for two pacemakers—at $4000 each. A billing error? I wonder how many of these billing errors have been omissions (undercharges) rather than overcharges. I'd bet not as many.

With the ongoing losses of tax monies that have been incurred by Medicare and Medicaid, Congress and the Health Care Financing Administration (HCFA, now CMS, the Center for Medicare and Medicaid Services) had the obligation to take some action. When it came out in the press in 2000 that Medicare had paid out $23 billion for billings that were not warranted, the story was presented in such a way as to criticize Medicare. Yet a grossly understaffed HCFA (or CMS)—it still has only about 4600 employees to oversee a program that pays out nearly $500 billion a year—did not have the resources to police such a huge nationwide program. Attacked by both sides—by the providers for having too many regulations and not reimbursing enough, and by Congress for reimbursing too much and not regulating enough—Medicare has come to be an example of "blaming the victim." Someone had to overbill or file fraudulent claims, thus ripping off Medicare and the American people. Those are the people who should be blamed, not Medicare.

Unfortunately, recent high-handed tactics by Medicare—with unfair, even Draconian legal and financial mandates—have embittered many providers. Combined with low reimbursement, these actions have led many physicians to stop seeing Medicare patients. Medicare is moving to change how it deals with physicians, to modify the high-handedness. Some limited legislation to improve the situation passed the House in December 2001, and more substantial legislative relief is being debated in Congress. Changes involving public policy often come slowly, as with most governmental actions. They require debate in a public arena, a disadvantage *and* advantage of a public (vs. private) system.

With the events of September 11, the public seems to have retreated a bit from the knee-jerk feeling that the private sector is always better than the public—or government—sector. At least with public safety, as with airport security, defense, police, and fire protection, the American public (and Congress, which voted for it) supports government solutions. Health care, like transportation, defense, and education, is an issue of vital public interest and safety (viz., the anthrax and smallpox threats). And good health is in the economic interest of the nation, not just the responsibility of each individual.

Expanding and Improving Medicare

MEDICARE WAS DESIGNED FOR 1965, and health care in America in the 21st Century has little resemblance to what it was then. Medicare needs to be improved and expanded. A concise summary explaining how this transformation could be accomplished is presented in a March 2001 "think piece" from the Economic Policy Institute.[2] However, there are powerful forces in America that are working against these kinds of changes. These special interests strive to maintain the status quo. Such is the case with the pharmaceutical industry, which reaps huge profits from the seniors who are forced to pay full price for their drugs. Or the insurance industry, which can make large profits by selling expensive MediGap policies or Medicare+Choice plans, which they can drop at will if they see their profitability threatened. Leaving their clients high and dry is no problem—not if the insurance company is losing money. And then there are the entrepreneurs, including the current administration and CMS Administrator Tom Scully, who would "reform" Medicare by privatizing it. It could be turned over to corporate America and transformed into a multi-tiered system where the rich would get one kind of care and the poor another kind.

I wonder if President Bush, Tom Scully, and other members of the current administration (and their supporters in Congress) are systematically trying to destroy Medicare by starving it financially. Such is the strategy that has been used in other countries, such as Canada and the United Kingdom, when conservative governments have tried to favor the private sector. The Bush administration could have been more aggressive in its efforts to roll back the 5.4 percent reduction in Medicare physician payments that occurred at the beginning of 2002 as a result of a faulty bureaucratic formula, but they didn't do it. And President Bush's projected budget allocations for Medicare (put out in March 2002) were woefully inadequate. As Paul Krugman noted in an op-ed piece in *The New York Times*, "...We have already reached the point at which we must either come up with more money or deny care to retirees...Medicare payments have already been squeezed beyond their limits, to the point where recipients can't find doctors willing to take them. Something will have to give, and soon."[3]

"Blaming the victim" (Medicare) plays to the interests of corporate America and enlists the support of an anti-government public bias that has been cultivated and nurtured by corporate and certain other political interests over the past two decades. Yet Medicare has demonstrated—at least for every American 65 years old and older—the feasibility of an equitable, theoretically affordable, and universal "safety net" for health care in America. There are very few seniors who would advocate for dismantling Medicare. So it's time Americans woke up, stopped "blaming the victim," and started protecting their safety net from those who would destroy it and leave those who are economically disadvantaged with secondor third-rate health care.

Americans could also start learning from the "Medicares," or national health insurance systems, of other countries, though many Americans seem to have an innate distrust of anything "foreign."

Summary of Key Points

- Medicare needs to be improved and expanded, not privatized or dismantled.

- National health insurance, with "one risk pool" for all Americans, similar to (an improved) Medicare, is *not* socialized medicine.

- "The government" is *not* an alien force. It is us.

Chapter 10

We Don't Want a Health Care System
Like They Have in Those Foreign Countries

"We have a health system that is the pride of the world."
— Professor David B. Williams[1]

"We're different from the other countries. I've heard say you're just a number there."
— A 65-year-old woman patient

MY WORK IN HEALTH care has taken me to 21 foreign countries, nearly all in the third world. I've also worked in Russia, which used to be categorized as "second world," but now might be better described as "otherworldly," at least with respect to its health care system. I've learned something about the health systems in other Western countries, especially Canada. I don't dare claim to be an expert on the European systems. However, I was once conned into giving a lunch presentation on the Scandinavian health systems at a meeting of Physicians for a National Health Program. I partially prepared for that talk by using a network of friends to get feedback via the Internet from Denmark and Norway.

Each developed country has its own unique system with its particular advantages and disadvantages. No system is perfect, and all of them are either currently experiencing financial problems or have had them recently. All are affected by politics. All have their critics and their defenders. And none of them are static. They all have been changing to reflect changing needs and changing economies. Some countries have experimented with privatization, usually under the aegis of conservative governments. So far, privatization has found a niche in several countries, but the trend has shifted back towards the strengthening of publicly funded services.

Every developed country—with the exception of the United States—has made a genuine effort to assure that every person living in that country has health care coverage (not just access). And, by and large, they have succeeded. No one in those countries has to worry about going without needed health care. It's true they may have to wait if the care is not urgent. In some cases, as in end-of-life situations, they may not receive heroic measures. But no one in those other countries has to worry about declaring bankruptcy because of their health care bills.

Even in the third world, where I have worked at a systems level for nearly 30 years, most countries recognize health care as a human right. Their constitutions include a right to health care. They have national public health systems, which act as a safety net for even the poorest people. Unfortunately, their ability to staff and supply their health care systems is often minimal.

The United States stands almost alone in the world in its failure to recognize health care as a human right. Instead we consider health care as an economic commodity. If you can afford it, you can get it. If not, you're out of luck—despite the myth that "anyone can go to the emergency room for care." Unfortunately, America is now exporting its market-driven philosophy of health care to other countries.[2] The effects could be disastrous for poor people in some of those countries, especially those in Latin America.

Considering that market-driven health care has been such a failure here, it's ironic, and sad, that we are selling our approach abroad. American corporations are trying to make profits abroad by encouraging the privatization of the parts of health sectors that offer potential for profit. Creating HMOs for the well-to-do. Diverting social security funds to private enterprise. The poor will be lucky to get the leftovers. And opposition to our "health care imperialism" may be stifled by trade agreements. The net results will likely be the raiding of social security funds in these countries and the further marginalization of the poor and their ability to get access to health care.

Americans Are Clueless
on What Happens in Other Countries

AMERICANS ARE GENERALLY UNINFORMED about what is happening in
other countries with respect to health care. They have no idea that
corporate America is actively exporting our profit-driven
approach to both industrialized and developing countries around
the world. And they are unaware that all the other industrialized
countries all spend much less than the U.S. on health care and yet
cover all their people. They don't know that:

a) We spend 50 percent or 70 percent more per person
   ($4200 vs. $2800 or $2400) on health care per person
   (1998 figures) than the next two most expensive countries (Switzerland and Germany, respectively), and 75
   percent more than Canada (which spends about $2300
   per person).[3]

b) Calculated as a percentage of GDP, U.S. health care
   spending is now about 40 percent more than the next
   most expensive nations—14.7 percent (a 2002 estimate)
   vs. about 10 percent.

Our excess expenditures for health care are despite—or
maybe partly *because of*—our failure to cover 15 percent of our
people. Indeed, Donald Light argues that universal access to
health care would greatly lower the overall cost of health care in
the U.S. It would grossly simplify our current complex systems
for billing, marketing, and administration—and save money. In
an article entitled, "Health Care for All. A Conservative Case,"
Light points out that our overhead (about 25 percent) is about
three times that spent in countries "with private care but universal access, such as Germany, Japan, and The Netherlands."[4]

The American public has pretty much bought into the myths
about foreign health care. These myths have been carefully
nurtured and financed by the special interests. The ingrained
myths include such oldies as (a) "We have the best health care
system in the world," (b) "They have rationing and waiting lines
in other countries," (c) "Why do so many people (especially

Canadians) come here for their health care?" No one, however, seems to boast about the Saudi royal family coming here for care. It doesn't have the same ring. Then there is the ever-useful slur (d) "They have socialized medicine," with the assumption that that must be bad, certainly un-American, and maybe even evil.

Per Capita Spending on Health Care – 1998

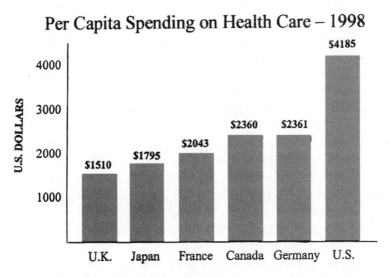

SOURCE: OECD. *Health Care at a Glance.* Paris. 2001.

Secondhand stories from friends or relatives in the other developed countries, notably Great Britain and Canada, tell mixed tales. Complaints about waiting lists for elective procedures, cancer treatment denied because someone was too old, controversial tabloid stories about emergency room disasters. There is an Idaho state senator who derides the Danish system for sending Danes to Mallorca in the winter for recovery and rehabilitation. I suspect it's cheaper, and more effective, to send people to recover in a warm climate than to keep them in a hospital in Denmark.

On the other hand, there are a host of stories that relate how far the systems in these other countries have gone to try to deliver the proper care. We hear of timely air evacuations in

Canada or coordinated holistic home care for the elderly in Great Britain. Maybe older Brits aren't as likely to get a kidney transplant when they're in renal failure. But they're much more likely than their American counterparts to have regular home visits to assess their overall needs from a team including a doctor, a nurse, and a social worker.[5] And ask Brits or Canadians if they'd like to switch their health care system for ours, as I have, and the reply will be overwhelmingly negative (of course, there always are some exceptions).

Americans who have had personal contact with health care systems in other developed countries tell about a variety of experiences. Sometimes they have encountered bureaucratic red tape, other times access has been simple. Their experiences have usually been favorable. They have generally been impressed with (a) the low cost of the care and (b) how much more humane the care seemed in comparison with America. An Idaho physician related how when he was in Ireland and suffered a mini-stroke, he had easy access to care, but they didn't have the expensive clot-dissolving drug to administer to him. My niece, who had her third baby in Dublin at about the same time, feels that her maternity care in Ireland was vastly superior to the care she had received in Washington, D.C.

In an article entitled "So Lucky to Give Birth in England," which appeared in a recent *New York Times* "Health and Fitness" section, an American woman who had a baby in London described her experience with the British system.[6] She subsequently had three more children in America. When friends ask her about her birthing experience in England, she tells them she "was lucky to be in London the first time around." Britain's National Health Service provided a daily home visit by a midwife for 10 days after the birth to check on mom and baby. She said that she "felt connected to a community, one that cared for its new babies and new mothers." With the birth of her last babies (twins) in New York City, she "was discharged within 48 hours and sent home to fend for [her]self."

David Burgess is a self-described American "right-winger" who works for *The Herald Tribune* in Paris. After receiving treatment for cancer of the esophagus in France, he wrote about his experience with the French health care system, and related how he had been converted to the merits of "socialized medicine." He wound up paying $6.50 out of pocket for medical care that an American physician friend told him would have cost over a half million dollars in the U.S. And Burgess praised the quality of care as excellent.

I've heard accounts from several Americans who were traveling abroad (specifically, stories from France, Spain, and Italy—as well as a personal one of my own from Switzerland). People relate how easy, and relatively inexpensive, it was to get care when they had an accident, usually a fracture. Some of them weren't even charged at all. And universally they note how they were treated with human kindness. That kind of caring happens in America too, but it seems to happen here with decreasing frequency. I hear in my mind the first question from the front desk, "Do you have insurance?"

Our Much-Maligned Neighbor to the North

CANADA, BECAUSE OF ITS proximity to the United States, has its own special spot in American mythology. They have long wait lists (not as much of a problem as it's presumed). It's socialized medicine (it isn't). Canadians are coming south "in droves"[7] for care (as opposed to the much larger number of Americans who go to Canada for cheaper medications or to have their babies). There are more CAT scanners in Peoria than in all of Canada (an exaggeration). Canadian ERs are falling apart under the demand (the same as in the U.S., it turns out). Canadian doctors are abandoning Canada to come to the U.S. (actual number about 500, or less than one percent of Canadian doctors, in 1999).

No one has disputed the quality of care in Canada—it's agreed to be at least equal to the quality in the U.S. And no one can legitimately complain about a lack of medical research in Canada. Canada produces at least as much research as does the U.S.—of course, in proportion to its population. Medical education in Canada is almost free, at least compared to the U.S., and graduates don't have $100,000 loans to pay off when they leave medical school. When they go into practice, they don't have the same incentives as their American counterparts to make money in order to repay a huge debt.

But Canada's system has born the brunt of negative advertising campaigns in the U.S., campaigns which have been successful in coloring Americans' perceptions of the Canadian system. The American Medical Association spent several million dollars in the early '90s to discredit the Canadian system and create doubts in the mind of the American public about a government-managed system for universal coverage. And in 2000, in a somewhat less successful ad campaign that cost perhaps $60 million, the American pharmaceutical industry tried to discredit the Canadian system. A ubiquitous "bus from Canada" appeared in a plethora of TV spots and full-page newspaper ads across the U.S. The goal was to derail efforts to make pharmaceutical benefits an integral part of Medicare.

Frank and Ernest

© 1995 Thaves / Reprinted with permission. Newspaper dist. by NEA, Inc.

The Canadian system has had its funding problems. They spend only a little over half as much per capita on health care as we do in the U.S., or about $2300 per person compared to $4200 per person in the U.S. (1998 figures). Or, in terms of percent of gross domestic product, Canada currently spends about 10 percent of its GDP on health, compared to 14.7 percent (2002 estimate) in the U.S. But despite problems with underfunding, the Canadians are able to cover every person with a fairly comprehensive health care package, which does vary from province to province as the system is not monolithic. And they are fiercely proud of their universal coverage. I remember a Toronto taxi driver (who had a foreign accent) holding up his medicare card and waving it proudly when we asked him about the Canadian health care system. "With this card I can get health care anywhere I want," he proclaimed.

Of course, there are Canadians who do complain. Complaining is a way to get change in Canada, as it should be in any democracy. However, if we were to compare the degree of seriousness of the complaints in Canada versus the U.S, it would be a "no contest." The U.S. "horror stories" would win hands down. There is much we could learn from Canada[8] if so many of us weren't so convinced that we had "the best health care system in the world." The other developed countries have learned a lot from each other, but we Americans automatically assume we have nothing to learn from the experience of others.

Our Ranking in the World

When we use objective criteria to compare our system to those of the other developed countries, we rank far from "best"— except in the area of spending, where we're way ahead of anyone else. As related above, the 2000 World Health Organization study that rated health systems of the world gave the U.S. 37th ranking in overall health system performance, a long way from number one. One can argue about the criteria that were used, but there's no doubt that in the category of "fairness," which played a heavy role in the rankings, we do very poorly. In fact, in the specific category of "fairness," we tied for 54th place with Fiji.

How about health outcomes? Our alleged "best health care system in the world," compared to other countries in the so-called "Health Care Olympics" of outcomes, consistently places 20th to 25th in criteria such as life expectancy, infant mortality, or immunization rates. The fact that we're by far number one in health care spending should raise some doubts about the value we Americans get for the amount of money we spend on health care. In all fairness, however, our poor showing for the standard health outcome measures is likely as much a result of America's wide social and economic disparities as our dysfunctional health care system. But given these wide disparities, the argument for universal coverage is even stronger.

We need to quit putting our collective heads in the sand as we blithely dismiss ideas from other nations, even the developing world. When I worked to help develop a primary health care system in Swaziland in 1989, we had an information system that gave us better data than I get in the U.S. today. Swaziland even had more options for birth control then because Depo-Provera was not yet being used in America. Yet because we assume we are "the best"—and have been encouraged to keep believing that assumption by the medical-industrial complex—we fail to look outside the U.S. for ideas. We need to acknowledge that our health care financing system is unfair, unjust, fragmented, expensive, wasteful, and broken. And that it behooves us to look north—and even south, west, and east—to learn how to improve our system so that it can be affordable and accessible to every person in America.

Summary of Key Points

- Americans are highly misinformed about the health care situation in other countries.

- America spends 50 to 200 percent more (per capita) for its health care than the other developed countries, yet, as a population, our outcomes are worse.

- All the other industrialized countries have universal coverage.

- America is the only developed country where getting sick or injured can, and all too frequently does, lead to bankruptcy.

PART TWO

Towards Finding a Solution

"We need to unite, get together, and demand universal coverage."

— A 62-year-old patient at my health center

Chapter 11

The Price of Health:
How Much Should We Americans
Be Spending on Health Care?

My wife's "Aunt" Selma relates how her long deceased husband, a pediatrician, used to help indigent patients back in the 1940s, when an office visit was $3. "He'd just take care of them and not worry about the payment. And he'd take care of patients at the free clinic and accept barter. That's the way it was."

WE'VE COME A LONG way since the Good Old Days, since the days when few people had (or needed to have) health insurance. Health care was a cottage industry. Most physicians were individual professionals practicing medicine as a labor of love and service. Medicine wasn't a bad living, but physicians—or for that matter, hospital administrators, many of whom were Catholic nuns—were not earning a fortune. Group practices, the few that existed, were reviled by the American Medical Association (AMA) as creeping socialism. General practitioners, like the fabled Marcus Welby, were icons in their communities. There were no expensive medicines or procedures. Nurses did nursing. Hospitals were mostly supported and run by communities or religious groups, not corporations. No one shunned "charity" care. It was a responsibility felt by almost every community and every physician.

In the early '40s, the charge for a physician's home delivery in rural Idaho was $40. Even in 1975, when I started an eight-year stint as a private solo-practice family doctor in Nampa,

Idaho, my charge for the regular office visit was $9. For a brief visit, it was $6.

In 1971, when I first became interested in health policy issues, the U.S. spent $70 billion a year on health care. That amount was then considered excessive, and Nixon's administration came up with the idea of promoting health maintenance organizations (HMOs), styled after the Kaiser plan, to control Medicare and Medicaid spending. In 2001, we had annual health expenditures of about $1.4 trillion—20 times as much (corrected for inflation, five times as much) and almost one-seventh of our total economy.

When I first opened my private practice in 1975, I decided (an economic gamble) to go without health insurance for my family and myself. We were young and healthy. And, at least in those days, physicians' fees for a doctor and his family were written off as medical courtesy. Economically, the gamble paid off. During the five years we were uninsured, I would have paid about $5000 for health insurance. And in those years we only incurred one expense of note. My eight-year-old son, attempting to simultaneously daydream and ride no-hands on his bike, fell and broke his arm. The fracture had to be set under general anesthesia. The hospital bill, including the operating room charge, came to about $300. The physicians, as was customary in those days, extended medical courtesy. Today, the operating room charges alone would be a few thousand dollars.

Although there is a small movement today by a handful of physicians and others (such as nurse practitioners) to set back the clock by practicing cut-rate cash-only ambulatory medicine, health care is no longer a cottage industry. The Good Old Days are long gone.

Of course, the Good Old Days weren't necessarily that good for everybody. For example, hospital workers were usually paid a minimum wage—in 1962, around $1 an hour. For them, that meant living in or near poverty. Medical interns and residents were paid $250 a month for a 120-hour workweek, a practice that persisted until they banded together in the mid-'60s to demand a living wage. When some interns applied for welfare, and qualified, the hospitals gave in. Then there were the pre-

Medicare days, when a great number of seniors stayed in poverty because of medical bills or simply went without medical care.

Medicare, after Social Security, became perhaps the most important solution to poverty for seniors. Medicare permitted retirees to live with dignity. Both Medicare and Medicaid made it possible for low-income elderly people and the poor to avoid becoming "health care beggars." Simultaneously, these programs helped support the hospitals and physicians who took care of them. Moreover, these two government programs led to social change. They mandated changes in civil rights like the desegregation of hospital wards. Prior to Medicare, in the early 1960s, the medical wards at the Johns Hopkins Hospital, where I trained, were segregated into separate floors for blacks and whites.

The "Good Old Days" Are Over

HEALTH CARE IN THE U.S. has long ceased to be a cottage industry. The change has been especially rapid over the past two decades. With rapidly rising costs and the squeezing of providers by managed care, financing health care for the uninsured has become progressively more problematic. Charity care, despite the barely measurable effect of "free clinics," has nearly vanished from the health care scene. To a great extent, so has the notion of "charity." Even for the insured, it can be a hard world. We saw an insured woman in her twenties with abdominal pain whom we referred to a surgeon for possible appendicitis. When she got to the surgeon's front desk, she was told she didn't have the proper referral forms required by her insurance company. She spent the next two hours crying in pain in her car in the parking lot. Luckily, she got better. It probably wasn't appendicitis.

The old practice of cost-shifting that allowed excess receipts from insured patients to cover the costs of the uninsured or indigent has largely disappeared. The excess receipts virtually evaporated or were pared down by (a) "Diagnosis Related Groups" (DRGs), where hospitals were paid by diagnosis, not cost, and (b) penny-pinching HMO contracts foisted on hospitals under the threat of losing their market share. However, with the recent collapse of managed care, the HMOs have lost much of their clout with the hospitals. It remains to be seen what will happen with charity care, but some hospitals, including our local hospital in Nampa, Idaho, have been more willing to write off some charges up front. Perhaps they realized they would be unable to collect anyway.

Specialists, meanwhile, have become less willing to write off the cost of consultations and procedures. Their business managers tell them they can't do it, and their front desks turn the uninsured patients away if they can't plunk down a large amount of cash up front. It has become increasingly difficult for cash-poor uninsured people to get specialist care. More recently, it has also become harder for cash-poor insured people to get the care they need because of the ever-increasing deductibles and co-pays. And if employers go in the direction of "defined contributions," as appears to be the case, such as with "personal health accounts," out-of-pocket health expenditures will only increase for employees.[1] The result will be that even middle-class insured Americans will find themselves in a more difficult bind.

Costs Are Going Up, Up, Up

A LARGE PART OF our current problem stems from the increasing cost of health care. As mentioned above, U.S. spending on health care went from about $70 billion in 1971 to $1.4 trillion in 2001. A recently released report from the Centers for Medicare and Medicaid Services (CMS) predicts that health care spending in the U.S. will double between 2002 and 2011–to a total of $2.8 trillion.[2] This would represent 17 percent of our GDP, compared to 13.2 percent in 2000. The per capita spending on health care in the U.S. would rise from $4637 in 2000 to $9216 in 2011. These figures represent an annual growth rate of 7.3 percent.

Premiums for health insurance are going up even faster. They increased by an average of 11 percent in 2001, and are expected to rise 15 percent in 2002. For 2003, CalPERS, the group that buys health insurance for California's public employees, and the second largest group purchaser of insurance in America, has accepted a 25.1 percent increase in premiums.

Some major factors responsible for the soaring costs of health care include an aging population, technological advances, increasing administrative costs, wasteful duplication of services, and an inflated pricing system. High consumer expectations, fueled by corporate advertising, media hype, and the Internet, also have contributed to the rising costs of health care, as has the cost of so-called "defensive medicine." But undoubtedly the most significant reason for skyrocketing costs has been new technology. A double-edged sword. While usually expensive, new technological advances have been both wonderful and incredible in terms of how they have affected our lives and our health. To list but a few examples of the positive effects of new technology:

- Joint replacements now allow older people to lead more fulfilling, less painful, and more active lives in their senior years.

- Bleeding or perforated ulcers, and their accompanying mortality, are now rare because of new medicines that suppress gastric acid secretion.

- Many operations are now much simpler, with less pain and much quicker recovery times, thanks to laparoscopic surgery and other microsurgical techniques.

- Intensive care for newborns that saves tiny premature babies—babies who only 25 years ago were left to die because they were considered too small to survive.

- Many heart attacks are now prevented by the placement of stents in narrowed coronary arteries.

- Many more people with mental illness can now be treated outside hospitals because of new, more effective antipsychotic and antidepressant medications.

Many of these advances, like the drugs that inhibit gastric acid secretion and have reduced the need for ulcer surgery, very likely have made health care *less* expensive. Blood chemistry panels have become incredibly *in*expensive—pennies a test—because of new techniques. But by vastly expanding the possibilities, new technologies have made medical care more expensive. In many cases, the technological advances (such as joint replacements) have made possible therapies that were unavailable in the past. A worn-out hip? In the old days, treatment might have been limited to a shot of cortisone and a walker. Do we need to return to those days because we can no longer afford to pay for hip replacements? Or should we consider saving $3000 by substituting a less-expensive artificial hip joint that only carries a five-year warranty?

Despite their cost, many of the new technologies offer some theoretical long-term savings. Joint replacements are effective in keeping the elderly out of nursing homes. The new "statin" drugs, though expensive themselves, will likely prevent millions of heart attacks and strokes, all of which are expensive to treat. However, the cost-benefit analyses for many of these new modalities usually don't show them to be cost saving in the "big picture." Sometimes the large number of interventions necessary to avoid a smaller number of catastrophes doesn't always balance out financially. For example, the universal administration of flu vaccine in the workplace has been shown to not be cost-effective. A failing of these cost/benefit studies, however, is that they usually do not factor in quality-of-life considerations. What is a week of good health without the flu worth?

A February 2002 study from the National Bureau of Economic Research by Yale economist William D. Nordhaus, however, suggested "the social productivity of health care spending might be many times that of other spending."[3] Maybe 17 percent of the GDP isn't too much. Nordhaus questioned the current feeling that our health care system is "stupendously wasteful" compared to other economic activities—at least when it comes to the overall benefits accrued to society. The finding is inherent in the nature of health care (it doesn't take an economist to appreciate the old adage that "if you don't have your health, you don't have anything"), but it doesn't excuse the internal wastefulness, injustice, and craziness of our current system.

Ethics—and Profits vs. Patients

BEYOND THE ISSUE OF pure cost, the new technologies have raised a host of ethical concerns. Cost is certainly a societal issue when we perform microsurgeries on babies' hearts inside the mother's uterus—at a cost of a half million dollars. Or when we save babies that weigh less than two pounds—at a cost of a few hundred thousand dollars. These same tiny babies have a high incidence of neurological damage later and require more resources. What about spending close to a million dollars (as the state of California is doing) for a heart transplant for a state prison inmate?

And how about our spending at the end of life? Should we be spending large sums of money in often-futile efforts to prolong life for the terminally ill elderly? End-of-life costs for medical care in America are considerable but often overstated. The actual estimate reflecting this cost is that 30 percent of Medicare spending goes to the beneficiaries of that program in their last year of life.

Where do we draw a line? Is that process called setting priorities—or rationing? When we didn't have the advanced technology, we did what we could as caregivers to alleviate pain and suffering. But now we must deal with the ethical issues involved with expensive measures such as bone marrow transplants, organ transplants, and other costly treatments for illnesses that cost hundreds of thousands of dollars or more. Some of the treatments have been shown to have questionable value, such as bone marrow transplants for breast cancer or extremely expensive antibiotics (a million dollars' worth) to treat Lyme disease.

The high-ticket items are the ones we usually hear debated. But, as any insurance actuary will tell you, these financial disasters are relatively rare. Including them in an insurance plan does not really add much to the cost of premiums—if there's a very large "risk pool." In contrast, the way clinicians practice everyday medicine involves hundreds of millions of patient encounters. And we clinicians are incredibly wasteful in our practice of everyday health care. A large part of the huge expense we incur is in excessive pricing. But much too large a part is in our failure to practice scientifically based medicine. Why should a young person with a first-time urinary tract infection be prescribed Cipro, which costs $100, when a $10 drug works just as well? Is it necessary that an echocardiogram (at $1200) be done for a healthy older person getting a cardiac evaluation? How often, and with what indications, should colonoscopy (at $2000) be done? What about liver biopsies (at $3000) for hepatitis C? Does every neck injury require an X-ray and/or a CAT scan? How many skin lesions (at $200 a whack) does the dermatologist really need to remove?

The conscientious (for some the word would be "zealous") specialist wants to be "complete." And she/he has a "stable" of costly procedures which (a) bring in good income and (b) make the patients feel they have been treated well. It's a three-part game of physician zeal (and, sometimes, greed), high patient expectations, and overpriced procedures/medications.

The "good part" of managed care was supposed to be about controlling these factors. But managed care got diverted into putting cost factors and profits first—despite the lip service to caring about people. As for practicing scientifically based medicine with a consideration for cost-effectiveness, America's health care is not yet there. Interestingly enough, some of the most practical work in using a scientific approach to diagnostic testing has come from Canada. The Canadians have developed objective guidelines, for example, to decide when and if X-rays are necessary for two common situations: ankle and neck injuries.

American researchers, such as the Agency for Health Research and Quality (AHRQ)[4] and the U.S. Preventive Services Task Force, are also busy developing guidelines. The latter entity applies a scientific approach to the analysis of preventive measures. Their recommendations are often critical of a host of costly, and even invasive, procedures advocated by some other groups. America's specialty groups, such as the surgeons, the gastroenterologists, and the gynecologists, tend to be more aggressive in their advice. Well-meaning as these specialists are, their viewpoint (often from a scope that gets threaded into a small orifice) might be called "narrow"—literally and figuratively.

How do we as a society decide what we will pay for? And how much are we willing to pay for those services?

Health policy expert Jonathan Weiner asserts that what America needs is "an accountable, transparent mechanism that makes use of scientific evidence, ethics, and consumer values to collectively decide what we can and cannot afford to cover as a basic insurance package."[5] For so-called "marginal" services, he adds, people could have optional coverage or pay out of pocket. He summarizes, "No industrialized nation spends more than America on medical care, excludes more of its citizens from coverage, and is less rational in the way it sets its spending priorities."

In the U.S., these financial choices have often been dictated more by politics and profits—or even happenstance—than by need. Why does Medicare automatically cover people with kidney dialysis? There must be hundreds of other conditions that deserve equal treatment. What about "Jerry's kids"? There is a host of other disorders that merit hoopla equal to that lavished upon muscular dystrophy. Yet periodically we are beseeched at the checkout stands of supermarkets and at street corners by well-meaning people collecting money for this specific, and relatively uncommon, ailment. Not to mention the telethons. American-style health care financing—and prioritizing.

"Expecting the World"

People in the U.S., at least if they have insurance, have come to "expect the world" from health care. How can you put a price on a child's life, especially if it's *your* child? How much is it worth to save a spouse who just had a heart attack? I no longer hear the kind of request I used to hear fairly frequently a decade or two ago, the request to "do everything possible—the cost doesn't matter"—to save 88-year-old grandpa. There has been a transformation in American society in our attitude towards death and dying, at least for the aged. I almost never see a living will now where an elderly person asks for extraordinary measures to preserve life. But it's totally different for younger folks.

People's expectations have been fueled and sustained by a corporate culture that has used "the market" to help create a society that "expects the world" from medical care. The sky's the limit from the new technologies—in terms of both an array of wonderful possibilities and (unfortunately) cost. Unlimited dreams, and unlimited profits, have helped create an American ethic, consistent with the free-enterprise spirit, that downplays the role of cost. Modern-day "snake oil merchants" are not only hawking an array of useful and not-always-so-useful products. They have also created a whole framework of myths and misinformation to assure their continued profits. And they have had huge influence over the media, which benefit financially from lavish spending on advertising.

This same corporate world has had a huge influence, through politics and lobbyists, on what direction American health care has taken. For the pharmaceutical industry, their campaign contributions and lobbying efforts have been rewarded with such perks as extended times for patents (e.g., Prilosec) and generous tax write-offs. The doctors (at least specialists) have managed to keep their fees high. And the insurance industry has (so far) been able to raise its premiums and exclude high-risk clients with little opposition.

As explained above, there was a brief period in the mid-1990s—in the heyday of the "managed-care revolution"—when the increase in health care costs seemed to flatten out. But at the end of the last decade, the HMO "bad guys" retreated. However, they could stage a comeback, as once again America is experiencing double-digit inflation in the cost of health care.

Did Americans really get what they wished for, as Princeton health economist Uwe Reinhardt has inferred?[6] Many Americans who bought into the expectation of health care without limits got tired of being restrained and abused by managed care. They helped make the HMOs back away from limiting care. Perhaps the HMOs, playing a competitive game that artificially lowered health care spending, realized that they could no longer profitably play the same game. They have been leaving Medicare managed care because the profits weren't there. Meanwhile, in all the maneuvering, they have not made patient interests a high priority. Leaving patients high and dry doesn't seem to matter, as the HMOs and insurance companies, like Aetna, seem to be starting to abandon the sinking ship of managed care, especially with regard to Medicare.

The Future, Technology, and Costs

THE HEALTH CARE INDUSTRY has largely played to the individual American's pursuit of personal happiness (with health, and all the trimmings). There has been little sense of responsibility to the community. In the Good Old Days, the center of most Americans' health care world was their general practitioner and their community hospital. Today, the focus has shifted to powerful insurance companies, mega-clinics, and giant HMOs, all of which have become increasingly for-profit. It's amazing how modern-day corporate health care has changed even the way Americans use language to frame the issues. It used to be that we had free choice of physician. Now we are told we need more choice of plan. And physicians didn't use to be "providers." It blows my mind to think that so many of us physicians have come to accept our being referred to as "providers" without throwing open our exam-room doors and shouting, "I'm mad as hell, and I'm not going to take this any more!"

The Good Old Days were when health care did not comprise one-seventh of the whole U.S. economy. Those days were before corporate America woke up and noticed that there was money to be made and fat to be trimmed in a sector of the economy that was huge and naïve to market forces. Health care had, and still has, the potential for a huge profit margin, as the pharmaceutical companies, the medical equipment manufacturers, and certain subspecialist physicians have learned.

There are still major market forces poised to "make a killing" in health care. The possibilities for profit coming from new technologies are immense. There is probably no other sector of the American economy that offers so much potential for profit. The American public has been primed for "endless health." They have become accustomed to having someone else pay for their health care. And they have been immunized against the forces of constraint, such as regulators and health care reformers, through the lobbying efforts and advertising campaigns of the medical-industrial establishment.

Will the ever-increasing spiral of health care costs ever end? At what point should it be slowed down or capped? What percentage of our GDP should be consumed by health care? Is 30 percent, a number some have predicted, too much?

An immediate danger of rising costs is the threat they present to the viability of Medicare and Medicaid. With a worsening economy, state and federal budget-watchers will have an excuse to gut these programs.

Some of our cost factors are clearly wasteful, illogical and exploitative. Pricing is crazy. There is an excess of administrative burden and waste. Our preoccupation with individual health and curative medicine has led us down the path of expensive cures when we should be investing much more in prevention, both on an individual and a societal basis. The path of prevention and community-centered health can be a force for lower costs, greater fairness and affordability. And, if we were to embrace universal coverage, we would reap further savings by largely eliminating delayed or omitted care, which lead to more serious and expensive interventions.

We can do nothing about the aging of our population, the greater number of elderly who will need health services. However, if our public health and preventive programs were effective, we could see people aging with fewer disabilities from chronic disease. There would be less heart disease, emphysema, diabetes, obesity, and joint disease secondary to obesity, etc. People wouldn't require as much expensive remedial care, like cardiac stents, bypass surgery, or joint replacements.

Prevention, specifically community-oriented prevention, is the path to choose. But prevention will have to compete for dollars with new technologies. And right now, the medical-industrial complex is putting its money on new technologies, not prevention. A paradigm shift toward prevention is in order (see Chapter 17).

David Callahan, in his book, *False Hopes. Why America's Quest for Perfect Health Is a Recipe for Failure,*[7] labels the new technologies and the medical paradigm of conquering disease and death as "false hopes." He supports the public health approach as well as the strengthening of our inner selves. I agree—and partially disagree.

Having experienced medicine in the age prior to our current wave of new technologies, I can say that I have seen some near-miracles in what some (but not all) of these advances have meant to people's lives. The 80-year-old woman who, facing invalidism in her final years, can suddenly play golf again with her new hip joint. Or the woman who avoided major surgery by having a cancerous polyp removed from her colon via colonoscopy. The hundreds of my patients who can live normal lives again because new, and more effective, antidepressants are available.

The new technologies hold great promise for the future, for future cures, and for prevention. If we could put at least as much money into developing new public health and preventive technologies, we would be better serving the interests of America. So I would agree with David Callahan that we should divert a good part of our investment from research on the expensive, limited-use technology to the kind of technologies that can benefit whole communities. It's common sense, not socialism.

What about those Americans who have either (a) relatively rare diseases, or (b) an ailment or injury that is very expensive to treat? Should they be denied the kind of advances that come with potential new technologies, like gene therapy? Should this new kind of technology be limited to the rich, who can pay for it with their own money?

Then there are the unfortunate people who have a combination of (a) and (b), a rare disease that is very expensive to treat. Such was the case of 19-year-old Brandy Stroeder (she has since died), an Oregon woman with cystic fibrosis who needed a heart/lung/liver transplant. The Oregon Health Plan, which covered her insurance, would not pay for the surgery she needed because "health plan officials argue[d] that the procedure is experimental and that funding must be reserved for primary and preventative services."[8] Oregon led the nation in trying to come up with a form of "rationing" of health care. For Oregon Medicaid patients, a list of diagnoses and treatments was drawn up with each item prioritized in order. Depending on available budget resources, a line is drawn on that list. The Oregon Health Plan reimburses items above that line. Below the line, the Plan won't cover it. Yes, it's rationing. And it was a methodology developed with careful and full community input. The reality is that, given limited public funds and unlimited technological advances, "rationing" of some sort is necessary—even in America, where "we don't want rationing." How should we Americans deal with the issue? What would have been the right decision for Brandy Stroeder?

The Answer Needs to Come From the People

I DON'T HAVE THE answer. But I feel the answer should come from the American people as a community. We should have the right as a community to decide where we put our pooled resources. Assuming we are well informed, and that is a large assumption, we should have input in deciding what projects should be researched by, e.g., our National Institutes of Health. If we decide as a community that we want to spend millions of dollars to seek a cure for a disease that only one of us has, because that's the kind of inclusiveness we feel as a community, then so be it. Or if we feel as a nation that we need to give more attention to researching alternative medicine, then we should be able to do that. If we decide that, as a community, we want to spend 30 percent of our GDP on health care (and, hopefully, public health and prevention get included), then that's okay. We'll have to spend less on other things. A recent article in the business section of *The New York Times*[9] raised the issue of whether health care should become the driver of the American economy. Goodbye General Motors and Exxon Mobil.

A major potential problem in expanding health care to such a huge percentage of our economy is the concern about getting value for our investment. If the history of health care costs to date is any measure of our success, we've failed. We've gotten poor value for our bucks. Unless we tie increased investment in our health care sector with a major paradigm shift to public health and prevention—and better outcomes—we'll be throwing away our money.

The problem with the community process for setting priorities is the likelihood of its being tainted by the vested health care interests and their myths. They have consistently used their influence, media campaigns, lobbyists, or campaign contributions to get the results they want, the results that will protect and enhance their financial interests. Given today's political reality, it may take some other very basic measures, such as campaign finance reform, to allow the community process to work. It will not be an easy task (see the following chapter) for Americans to win meaningful health care reform and affordable health care with such a powerful array of corporate interests blocking the way.

Meanwhile, if we are to prioritize some expensive new technologies, how about an artificial heart for the insurance industry? Maybe then, they'd care about us.

Summary of Key Points

- The cost of America's health care continues to escalate at a rate considerably above the rate of inflation.

- New technologies are the major factor driving the higher costs even as they make some interventions more affordable.

- We get poor value in America for the money we spend on health care.

- With our escalating costs, we need to invest a much greater proportion of our health care dollars in prevention and public health.

- As a nation, we need to make our expectations more consistent with how much we are willing to spend on health care vs. other expenditures.

- Health care has the potential to become "the driver" of our economy.

Don Quixote vs. the Establishment: Can the Medical-Industrial Complex Be Toppled?

On the cover of the December 9, 2001, Chicago Tribune *Magazine is a full-page color photo of a thoughtful-appearing Quentin Young, MD. Large letters across the picture read "Doc Quixote." The subscript: "For 50 years, Quentin Young has pushed for health care for all. Will he ever realize his dream?"*

"The [health care] system is controlled by a small handful of powerful people, economic forces, whose profit-making takes precedence over the national, and indeed, the world cause of good health."[1]
— Rep. John Conyers, (D-MI)

MOVED BY A DESIRE to improve access to health care in America, in 1990 I decided to run for the Idaho State Legislature. As a result, some of my colleagues compared me to Don Quixote tilting at windmills. Years later, I reflected upon those windmills as I rode past a huge complex of hospitals near downtown Denver. I gazed with awe at the large illuminated signs on the sides of the towering buildings. These guys are big, rich, and powerful. And they have powerful friends and allies, like the insurance companies, the pharmaceutical industry, and organized medicine. They can drop a few million dollars to try to kill a ballot initiative in California or Massachusetts—or a referendum in Portland, Maine. Against such odds, how much chance did I have to shake up the "medical-industrial complex"? The forces to oppose change control one-seventh of our economy. And there I was, gazing up at these huge monoliths of power. Don Quixote. A community health center physician serving mostly low-wage uninsured patients who pay a $10 nominal fee for a visit. Fortunately Quentin Young, and others like him, are on our side.

Health care in America has evolved into an incredibly complex entity. Our system is so fragmented and complicated that it's almost impossible to comprehend. It's easy to plant doubt ("There must be a better way") in the public mind, doubt that will make people wary of change. It's also easy, when you have lots of money, to create and perpetuate myths that protect the status quo. In the face of such powerful opposition, what can we Don Quixotes do to fix our fragmented, costly, and inequitable system, a system that excludes one-seventh of our population from adequate access to care? Can we do something to improve our dismal near-to-last ranking among the developed countries for almost every health indicator?

"The Evil Empire": How Bad Is It?

THE U.S. DEPARTMENT OF Health and Human Services has an initiative, "Zero Disparities," linked to *Healthy People 2010*, to eliminate all health care disparities. It's extremely unlikely to happen unless America has universal coverage. To quote Rep. Donna Christian-Christensen (D-VI), "There can be no elimination of disparities if everyone...does not have insurance coverage."[2] And America will never have meaningful or affordable universal coverage as long as the powerful vested interests hold sway over what happens to health care in America. The uninsured and the folks on the low end of the disparity gulf have probably less than one-tenth of one percent of the lobbying resources available to the "Gang of Four" (pharmaceutical industry, insurance industry, hospitals, and organized medicine) that comprises "the Evil Empire" of health care. The combined campaign contributions of health care's "Gang of Four" are unrivaled.

Incidentally, when I use the term "Evil Empire," I am by no means implying that the people associated with these groups are bad. The overwhelming majority of the people working for the "Gang of Four" are sincere, well-meaning, good people. They're just clueless. They're caught up in the complexity of the system and unaware of the disastrous effects their business dealings are having upon many millions of Americans. They have little appreciation that their quest for "market share" and healthy bottom lines is making "health care beggars" out of millions of Americans and robbing them of their dignity.

What's really wrong is the value system that we have come to accept as a society. It's a value system that has helped create—and sustain—"the Evil Empire." It might be called the "Enron" paradigm. Push the legal envelope in the name of free enterprise. If you occasionally cross to the wrong side of the legal system, you pay your fines and continue on. Unless you're an Enron and go bankrupt, of course. It doesn't matter how many people are hurt in the process. If millions must go without heat or air conditioning because energy prices soar, and a few older folks die in the process, well, that's "the market." And the government will find some temporary solution to deal with the people who are most vulnerable, right?

Health care poses a similar situation. The parallel is uncanny. Millions go without health care because they can't afford it. People die because they delay care. And an ethic sanitizes the process by asserting, "That's just the effect of 'the market.'" Profits before patients because we believe in free enterprise, and, in the long run, "the market" will solve the problem. "Personal responsibility" for the consumer, but the primacy of self-interest for the "Gang of Four." Lip service to universal coverage (it sounds altruistic) but keep the status quo so our bottom line isn't threatened. That's hypocrisy.

But it's worse. "The Evil Empire" has its plotters and their henchmen. They're not quite the same as the out-and-out crooks who use electronic chicanery to collect on services that were never delivered to patients. But it's sort of like "soft" porn. Overbilling for home health services. Systematic up-coding of diagnoses so third-party payers will pay more for services. Rationalizing expensive procedures or surgeries for patients who don't really need them. Using "creative accounting" to write off marketing expenses as health education. Lobbying legislators to push agendas that are shady. Writing legislation for them that protects practices that are marginal but profitable. The list goes on. The captains of industry begin to look more and more like pirates. And our society either (a) accepts all this highway robbery as "part of business as usual," or (b) is totally clueless. Unfortunately, both apply.

We modern-day Don Quixotes, like Quentin Young, have realized that the system is broken and corrupt. And what we're basically fighting, like Cervantes' Don Quixote, is a whole culture. We're committed to a similar quest, righting a wrong that too few around us perceive to be wrong. Our information system today is a little more sophisticated than the 17th century novel. It's easier to get our word out. But it's also easier for the Gang of Four to buy a few million dollars of media time to cloud the issue. Or to make sure that symposia and proposals that deal with getting to universal coverage include poison pills—e.g., "must be pluralistic"—that protect the status quo.

Toppling the Windmills

PERPETUATING THE CURRENT COMPLEX system clearly fits the financial interests of the Gang of Four, or so they think. It allows them the potential to find opportunities for profit by manipulating the system. There are exceptions, some industry players who haven't totally forgotten about the needs of patients. But, generally speaking, as America's health care system has evolved, patient interests have largely been secondary to financial and business interests.

If we were to have comprehensive reform that had universal coverage with "one risk pool" and affordable, comprehensive care, the Gang of Four could be adversely affected financially. For starters, the pharmaceutical companies would be subject to group purchasing. Their worst nightmare, even beyond pharmaceutical benefits becoming an integral part of Medicare, would be to have all Americans covered with one risk pool. Either way, group purchasing power could cut their profits in half, or there could be price controls for drugs. As for the insurance companies, their cut of the health care pie, which now provides them with hefty commissions and profits, would be almost eliminated. They would be relegated to administrative duties, much as they do with Medicare today.

For physicians, medical subspecialists could see their incomes drop. There would be pressure to have more realistic pricing for their services. The historical over-reimbursement for medical and surgical procedures would change. As for the hospitals, the for-profits would need to worry about reduced bottom lines or convert to not-for-profit status. All hospitals, however, should welcome change that would help cover the costs of the uninsured patients they currently care for anyway.

I remember when a small group of people (including myself) from an organization that was then called the Idaho Citizens' Network put together a single-payer universal coverage health care reform bill for Idaho in 1991. We even managed to get an Idaho state senator to sponsor it and introduce the plan, called "IdaHealth," as legislation. A few people still kid me about how the bill failed in the Senate by a vote of 42–0. But when it came out, it caused a mild panic among the leaders of the health establishment. Fax machines (this was in the days before e-mail) fairly burned up in the establishment's quest to get the word out to defeat the plan.

In my idealistic and naïve hopes, as a (then) member of the Board of Trustees of the Idaho Medical Association, I tried to convince my fellow trustees (at least) not to oppose the legislation. Fat chance. It wasn't particularly difficult to get the Medical Association to endorse universal coverage as a concept (words are easy and cheap), but an actual bill was too much of a threat. The old war cry of "socialized medicine" rang out, and some physician friends referred to me as "their favorite communist."

What will it take to knock down the windmills? Actually, unless we have some cataclysmic event (and September 11 comes close), I don't think we Don Quixotes have much of a chance to defeat the forces of the "Gang of Four"—at least not by any frontal attack. The arguments for health care as a right, social justice, or compassion will continue to be countered by well-meaning (though sometimes greedy) people who will argue for "personal responsibility," market solutions, and for-profit schemes disguised as "more choice." The events of September 11 and the subsequent fear (and reality) of bioterrorism have created some heightened sense of community in America. The tragedy also may have mitigated the tendency for many Americans to espouse the ideals of "everyone for himself"—or, in the health care rhetoric, "personal responsibility." But idealism is probably not the "silver bullet" for meaningful reform. Economics most likely is.

Appealing to Self-Interest— Does It Have a Chance?

APPEALING TO THE CONSCIENCES of the Gang of Four will probably do little to eliminate the windmills, though it's certainly important to have a strong philosophical basis to support the reasons for health care reform. And it's key that we have a widespread grass-roots effort to try to weave the principles of social justice into the fabric of the American psyche. A more fruitful approach might be to convince the Gang of Four to voluntarily dismantle the windmills, to make them see that it would be to the advantage of not only the American people, but also in their own economic interest, to embrace universal coverage.

Seemingly, it would be difficult to convince the insurance companies to (in effect) self-destruct. It could mean shutting their doors and laying off many of their 1.3 million employees. Yet, as the cost of health care increases exponentially and health insurance becomes increasingly unaffordable, insurance companies may want to get out of "risk" situations in health care. They could shift their role and become contract administrators for a national health plan. They would get their cut of the payments. And they could avoid potential losses, the kinds of losses suffered by about half of the for-profit HMOs in the waning days of the managed-care bubble. They could voluntarily choose to get out of the "risk" business.

The Drug Barons

THE PHARMACEUTICAL COMPANIES WILL fight fiercely to defend their
windmills. They owe it to their stockholders. However, under
pressure, they have been retreating in a few areas. On the international front, they reduced their prices on drugs used for
HIV/AIDS. They even offered to donate the drugs. But their
capitulation only came after years of maintaining high prices for
everyone. They gave in only when it was apparent that cheaper
generic versions of the drugs would come from India or Brazil.
The drug companies have tried to sweeten their own image with
charity-type programs in the U.S., like Pfizer's "Sharing the
Care" program in community health centers, including ours.
Pfizer and other pharmaceutical companies have now come out
with a low-cost (in Pfizer's case, $15 a drug) prescription offer
for low-income Americans—likely a response to the hullabaloo
raised by windmill chasers. These programs do help low-income
people, and they cost the drug companies almost nothing. The
people affected would have been unable to afford the medicines
anyway. Meanwhile, the pharmaceutical companies earn brand
loyalty from the clinicians who prescribe their drugs.

In the big picture, the pharmaceutical industry will fight
to retain its profits since that is their primary mission. Some
analysts argue that if we had national health insurance (NHI), the
drug companies' profits wouldn't necessarily drop. They would
in theory make up in volume what they lose by cutting prices. In
the long run, the U.S. will undoubtedly adopt price controls for
drugs, just as every other developed country has done. At some
point, our leaders will realize that it is in the greater interest of
our nation to have access to effective and affordable care than to
sustain a specific industry at a rate of profit margin way in excess
of any other industry.

The rhetoric (1) that the pharmaceutical industry needs its
huge profit margin for research and development, and (2) that
drugs have to be more expensive in the U.S. because American
companies do the lion's share of developing new drugs, is myth
and rubbish (see Chapter 1, Myth #11). They've got a good deal
going, and who can blame them for wanting to keep it working

for them? They will fight the battle to maximize their profits until they see the writing on the wall that says "price controls." Maybe then they will voluntarily come over to the side of NHI.

The Camelots of Health Care

DESPITE THE RECENT PROLIFERATION of for-profit hospitals, most hospitals have the interest of their communities in mind. But the field of inpatient care has changed in recent years. It has become a much more diverse entity. Nursing homes, which used to be mostly community-based, have now largely been converted to for-profit, chain ownership. Much of what used to be done as inpatient care has now been converted to outpatient care at ambulatory care centers. These have been largely for-profit entities. They attract the paying patients and procedures. Thus, they have left the hospitals with a greater share of the uncompensated care. And the hospitals cannot turn away (or refuse to admit) patients who walk into their ERs—including the uninsured. From a fiscal standpoint, the hospitals should support NHI.

Unfortunately, the hospitals' experience with Medicare has often been unfavorable and frustrating. When I advocate for an improved and expanded Medicare for All, many hospital administrators roll their eyes. They've been so stressed out with dealing with Medicare's bureaucratic demands that they worry about having more of "such a good thing." Depending on their Medicare/managed-care mix, hospitals may in alternate years complain about how their private-sector payments must subsidize Medicare, or vice versa. But they will admit that the managed-care bureaucratic burdens are often worse than Medicare's. And the prospect of having only one insurance payer with one set of forms and rules does provide a measure of hope for the hospitals. Their administrative burdens could be vastly simplified.

In the old days, Medicare just paid the hospital's bill, no strings attached. But since the initiation of DRGs (Diagnosis Related Groups, or where Medicare pays a hospital by diagnosis, no matter how long the patient stays in the hospital), and other bureaucratic demands, hospitals have been much more wary of Medicare. The hospitals, especially the for-profits, brought much of this added red tape on themselves. Medicare fraud, like the fraudulent up-coding done systematically by HCA/Columbia, precipitated the tightening of the screws. "Improving" Medicare means making it simpler. But we also need to expect a greater degree of honesty on the part of health care providers. This honesty will be difficult to achieve without removing incentives to maximize shareholder profits. The for-profits will be difficult to convince. Maybe they should be converted to a not-for-profit status so we once again have "a level playing field" in health care. Not-for-profit hospitals should have every reason to support NHI since they would no longer have to write off their services to uninsured patients as uncompensated care.

The Lords of Medicine

THE PHYSICIANS ARE A mixed bag. A large number of physicians of all specialties (especially primary care doctors and psychiatrists) actually support single-payer universal coverage. Physicians for a National Health Program (PNHP), an organization started in 1987 to promote single-payer national health insurance, has over 9000 members. However, many physicians underestimate how much their colleagues support NHI, as a recent study showed. In a national survey of medical school faculty, residents and students, published in the *New England Journal of Medicine* in 1999, 57 percent chose single payer as the best solution for America's health care ills.[3] However, the medical establishment, as represented by the American Medical Association (AMA), has been staunchly against single-payer universal coverage. Fearing a Canadian-style health care system, the AMA spent millions of dollars in the early '90s to finance an advertising campaign of disinformation aimed at discrediting Canada's system of universal coverage. The AMA prefers system changes that, bluntly described, would protect and increase physicians' income and autonomy. Their solution stresses "personal responsibility" and patient "choice" (with the physician still in the driver's seat) through constructs such as medical savings accounts (MSAs) and tax credits.

It amazes me how generally ignorant many, if not most, physicians are about how our health care system works—or doesn't work. Some may be motivated by their own narrow economic interests, but many do care about improving access to health care. Yet they have no idea of the larger picture, especially from their patients' viewpoint. Despite spending long hours buried in the everyday work of their profession, most physicians remain "technicians." They have little appreciation of the difficulties faced by the uninsured and (now) underinsured. They are simply too busy, too tied up in their daily chaos, to take notice of what is really happening to their patients. More poignantly, they are even more unaware of the patients they never see. Those are the uninsured patients who (a) come in but aren't seen because they lack the $200 they're asked to plunk down at the front desk, or (b) don't even bother to come in because they don't have the cash in hand and have too much pride to be rebuffed by the receptionist.

The physicians—as well as other health care professionals— should be much easier to convince to tear down the windmills. In fact, many professional organizations have been actively coming up with proposals for universal coverage, some of them quite progressive (beyond such narrow solutions as MSAs). Some of the proposed plans have even been really "universal," such as the proposal being put forward by the American Academy of Family Physicians (AAFP). Their plan calls for (in effect) single-payer universal coverage for primary care, prevention, and catastrophic costs. Their original draft even excluded deductibles and co-payments, though they reinstated the co-payments in the final version. The AAFP plan advocates tax-based financing as well as separation of employers from the purchasing of health insurance. What a long way physicians have come.

It remains unlikely that the Mother of all American medical associations (the AMA), with its long history of largely success-ful opposition to national health insurance—they helped derail every plan in the 20th century—will support any meaningful solution. But the AMA is losing its influence as the other medical organizations take leadership on this vital issue. There is hope. Physicians are increasingly discussing universal coverage.

It's only a matter of time until they realize the need for an affordable, equitable solution that embraces national health insurance.

Tilting at Windmills From Beyond the Medical Establishment

THERE ARE OPPORTUNITIES OUTSIDE the "Gang of Four" to do battle with the windmills. Perhaps the most promising hope for action comes from convincing the American business community that national health insurance (NHI) would be in their economic self-interest (see Chapter 3). It's evident that NHI would also be in the best interest of their employees. It would be a way to break the perverse and increasingly onerous link between employment and health insurance. The link developed as a fluke of history. During World War II wage controls froze workers' pay, so employers began to offer employees health insurance as an extra benefit. No other developed country has this anachronistic mechanism. Nonetheless, recent surveys show that a large majority of the American public is satisfied with the employer-based system. Perhaps the respondents were unaware of other options, but their comfort with the current system illustrates how difficult it may be to convince Americans that a change would be to their advantage.

The time is quickly approaching, however, when business will have to take a hard look at how it is providing health insurance for employees. The impetus behind the managed-care revolution of a decade ago came from business. Under economic siege from rapidly escalating health insurance costs, business led the change to managed-care plans to control runaway costs. The "fix" was temporary, and health insurance costs are again increasing at double-digit rates. Employers have already been shifting costs to employees with ever increasing co-pays and deductibles. And employees are starting to hurt more as they join the swelling ranks of the "underinsured." Now employers are looking toward "personal health accounts" and "defined-contribution" approaches, euphemisms for further shifting the costs to employees. The effect would be to cut loose the employees' security lines in a wild sea of increasing premiums for health insurance.

For a while, not so long ago when the unemployment rate was low, some employers regarded the health insurance benefit as a recruitment and retention tool. But with a rising unemployment rate, this factor is no longer so important. Employers are likely to wake up soon, see the light at the end of the tunnel, and shed their health insurance relationship with their employees. It makes economic sense—especially in a global market where competing corporations in other nations are not saddled with this albatross of a cost. Employees will experience a progressively more difficult time in navigating an increasingly expensive and perilous health insurance market. If they should be so unfortunate as to have a preexisting condition, they will be even worse off. The obvious affordable and practical solution would be automatic universal coverage with a single risk pool. Business has to wake up soon, if for no other reason than out of economic self-interest. And when business speaks, America and American politicians listen.

There are new opportunities for windmill bashing since 9/11. Compared to a sense of community, "personal responsibility"—everyone for himself—doesn't seem to be quite as important as it used to be. Out of the disaster has come a feeling that we're a community, that we have some shared responsibility for each other. Even "government" seems to have gained some stature. In an October 2001 *New York Times* op-ed piece, Robert Putnam, author of *Bowling Alone: The Collapse and Revival of American Community,* opined that the new sense of community would not be short-lived. He concluded that, "This new period of crisis can make real to us and our children the value of deeper community connections."[4] In addition, there's the whole new dilemma of what we do for victims of bioterrorism. A special fund? New complex eligibility rules to access the fund? Everyone for himself? Out of 9/11, there's new hope for universal coverage. The "we're all in this together" argument has a new validity that more Americans can now appreciate.

If we can pull together enough Don Quixotes, we can create a large enough grassroots movement to demand change because "we're all in this together." As an inveterate Don Q. myself, I'd like to deputize every man, woman, and child in America for the cause. Maybe then the medical-industrial complex would be forced to capitulate, to realize that the interests of America as a whole will be better served if we have universal coverage. And, as a true dreamer, I'm campaigning for 100 percent, not 92 or 95 percent, because the forgotten 5 or 8 percent are bound to be my patients. They're the ones most likely to fall between the cracks because, (a) they don't have the means to negotiate a ridiculously complex system, or (b) they have conditions that make them health insurance pariahs.

Most thoughtful people, including business and corporate gurus, who have lived with our dysfunctional nonsystem for decades admit that America eventually will have to go to some type of national health insurance. Many even use the words single payer. The windmills will fall. I hope it will be sooner rather than later. The sooner it comes, the less the disenfranchised—those without adequate access to timely care—will have to suffer needless anguish and misery. Meanwhile, we are likely to pursue a variety of partial fixes or piecemeal approaches as we attempt to find "a uniquely American" solution. Doc Quixote will realize his dream—some day. And it will take a grassroots approach to get there.

Summary of Key Points

- It's likely that some sectors of the medical-industrial complex will see an advantage to universal coverage with national health insurance. Undoubtedly some will not, and the struggle will not be easy.

- As they have become more informed, physicians have increasingly become more favorably disposed towards universal coverage.

- Businesses need to wake up and realize that their current role in purchasing health insurance is not only outdated but also puts them at a competitive disadvantage with their counterparts in other countries.

- It will take a grassroots effort to change our system, but the system will change eventually.

DR. SPRECHER'S
PITTSBURG ELECTRICAL INSTITUTE
308 PENN AVENUE.
All Chronic Diseases cured by Electricity.

Chapter 13

In Search of a "Uniquely American" Solution to Health Care for All

"We need a pragmatic, not an ideological solution. Reduce the number [of uninsured Americans] *from 39 million to its irreducible minimum, probably about 15 million, and consider that a victory and not a terrible tragedy."*
— Dr. Richard Corlin, president of the AMA, speaking in Cedar Rapids, IA, April 2002[1]

IN MY WORK AS a physician at a "safety-net" clinic, I am aware on a daily basis of the problems faced by the uninsured and, now increasingly, the underinsured.

The conventional wisdom of our health industry gurus and our political leaders tells us that, to solve our uniquely American problems with health care, we will need a uniquely American solution. Of course, we are already unique in many ways. We're the only developed country without universal coverage. We're unique in how we so closely tie health insurance to employment. We're unique in having such a high proportion of personal bankruptcies—almost 50 percent—tied to medical bills. We also may be unique in our ability to get so little value for the huge amount of money we spend on health care. British, French, Cuban, or Canadian solutions will not do.

The issues are complex. Health care organization is not simple. Multiple solutions proposed over the past 90 years have been shot down,[2] deemed either impossible, unworkable, overly bureaucratic, too dependent on government, too expensive, or simply unacceptable to the American public.

Unfortunately, the direction we appear to be headed could lead to "health care meltdown." We're becoming more of a multi-tiered system that progressively excludes the poor and the sick, and soon (if not already) the middle class as well. Piecemeal approaches with increased complexity—such as tax credits, vouchers, "defined contributions" with managed care, medical savings accounts, and personal health accounts—will only result in more holes for people to fall through, more delayed care. A few may benefit, but many will be harmed. Why not consider simplifying the system?

Perhaps we need to "think outside of the box," consider an alternative, which should garner support as the antithesis of "socialized medicine." Why not consider an approach which would maximize the American value of "personal responsibility," level the playing field, and be truly universal in nature? How about considering, as an intellectual exercise, an approach that reflects the logical (and absurd) endpoint of present-day conservative thinking in America, a "uniquely American" solution: universal uninsurance.

Universal Uninsurance

DO AWAY WITH ALL health insurance. Abolish it completely. Allow free exercise of our ability to be creative and entrepreneurial. We could remold our health care system using the American values of rugged individualism, personal responsibility, belief in the free market, and—not to be forgotten—compassion for our neighbors.

Eliminating bureaucracies like Medicare, Medicaid, HMOs, and health insurance companies would save billions of dollars. Employers would be relieved of the burden of providing health insurance for their workers. Employees would get larger pay-checks instead of having their hard-earned wages diverted to ever more expensive health insurance plans with increasingly shrinking benefits. People would be forced to care about the cost of their health care. Managed care would be gone. No longer would we have messy, unfair, and resource-wasting government regulations or restraints on utilization and referrals. Two hours on the phone to get a procedure approved?

American technology would form part of the solution. Consumers would be incentivized to make much greater use of the Internet for health information. In true American style we could have huge health care mega-malls, like Wal-Health or Health Depot. Shopping centers could offer a wide range of practitioners including alternative medicine. Blue light specials. Coupons to clip in the Sunday papers for discounts on colon cancer screening. Half-price purple pills (flown in from Mexico). The possibilities are limitless.

What About Poor Folks?
Charity Care to the Rescue

BUT WHAT WOULD HAPPEN to poor folks? The people without even enough money to buy the Sunday paper to clip the coupons? Or the homeless folks without a mailing address to receive the junk mail with money-saving health care specials?

We will look to our past and the great American tradition of charity care. Physicians who are nostalgia buffs will be overjoyed to be able once again to offer free care to the needy. Freed up from the bare-bones payments of managed-care plans and Medicaid, physicians will be able to afford giving charity care. Hospitals will again have the capacity to cost shift.

Compassion could flourish. After all, compassion, as in "compassionate conservatism," is part of the American way of being. Poor folks will once again be able to feel grateful for the free or reduced-price care they receive. It will be individuals helping individuals, not the government butting in. We will be able to circumvent the whole messy philosophic argument about health care being a human right.

There could be a profusion of free clinics. The plethora of bored specialists who retired early to escape managed care could volunteer to work in free clinics. For people too proud to use the services of free clinics, but still unable to afford needed health care, there could be a host of pluralistic solutions for financing their care. Americans love pluralistic solutions—and choice—or so we're told. Some tried-and-true American solutions for financing health care for individuals in need:

- The bake sale. Selling only 1000 three-layer chocolate cakes at $8.99 each could finance a gallbladder operation, if the beneficiary only stayed in the hospital one day. For those who might be interested in extending this model on a nationwide scale: if each person in America sold just one nine-inch German chocolate cake a day at $9.99 apiece, the proceeds (one trillion dollars) would be enough to cover 100 percent of America's health care costs, assuming administrative savings from eliminating insurance. There would also be a grand opportunity for choice/pluralism: we could sell apple pies, peach cobbler, cherry cheesecake, etc. The possibilities are limitless.

Health Care Financing – and Choice – U.S. Style

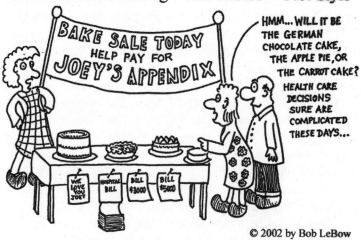

© 2002 by Bob LeBow

- Coin boxes at supermarket checkout stands and self-service gas stations to collect money for, e.g., Sammy's hernia repair, or Max's Viagra.

- Lotteries or Bingo games set up on an ad-hoc basis to meet the crisis health care needs of a needy individual.

- To raise money for expensive procedures, an array of other activities such as concerts, telethons, phone cards, car washes, donating the cost of a meal not eaten, mowing lawns, etc. (Columnist Molly Ivins relates "there are more than 1000 concerts given every week by musicians for other musicians to raise money for an operation or medical treatment of some kind.")[3]

These types of activities, like holding a raffle to pay for an emergency appendectomy, provide great opportunities for building cohesiveness in a community. In fact, if communities elect to go even further, they could come up with community-based approaches to health care financing. Catastrophic funds, hospital taxing districts, local sales taxes for health, sin taxes, and the use of tobacco funds are but a few of the innovative ways in which communities could respond to the need. Charitable foundations and religious organizations could supplement these funds.

Perhaps the most attractive aspect of universal uninsurance is the level to which it raises the importance of "personal responsibility." It's almost like the TV game of "Survival."

Potential Obstacles to Universal Uninsurance

WHAT ABOUT PEOPLE WITH Medicare? Wouldn't they oppose this approach? Most would probably support the change once they realized that Medicare is in fact a government program. Others would need to be convinced that it was the American way, that it wasn't proper for America to have a health care system that looked anything like those other countries' socialized medicine.

And what about people who might be inclined to buy insurance to protect themselves from financial ruin? The nonbelievers who are skeptical of "bake-sale" financing? They would need to be convinced that their sentiments were un-American, perhaps even unpatriotic. They would need to renew their faith in "the market."

Of course, it's unlikely that pure universal uninsurance could ever become a reality in America. As a colleague told me, Americans are hesitant to support "one size fits all." Even more significantly, the insurance companies, hospitals, and pharmaceutical industry would all oppose it. Demand could evaporate for the $1000 toenail fungus treatment that people read about in the Sunday supplements. They could no longer demand the product "because their insurance paid for it." Sales of $80 a month Clarinex might drop when people realized they could buy a generic drug with equivalent efficacy for two dollars a month. And health insurers would obviously be out of business. Employers might even oppose it, as employees would likely have more freedom to change jobs, just as they would with the diametrically opposite approach to health care reform, national health insurance.

The Sad Truth: Fantasy May Resemble Reality

IT'S UNCANNY, HOWEVER, HOW much this tongue-in-cheek spoof I have described on universal uninsurance resembles reality. It's a direction in which American health care could be headed. A game of "Survival"—even for the middle class. There are even some people, like the members of a basically libertarian organization called the American Association of Physicians and Surgeons, who could actually support the universal uninsurance fantasy as I've described it.

The newest maneuvers *du jour* to control costs (for employers, but not employees) are scary in their resemblance to universal uninsurance. Business interests seem to be heading in the direction of a "defined-contribution" approach. This strategy in effect caps employer spending for health insurance and shifts costs—and risk—to employees. It's like the model outlined above with a fixed employer contribution thrown in. For someone who has a chronic illness or who gets sick or is injured, "defined contribution" is like a crapshoot. And it does nothing to address the problem of the uninsured.

Promoters of the "defined-contribution" approach have dressed up the idea by terming it "consumer-driven" health care, when it's really "risk-assumed-by-employee" health care. Extolling the myth of "more choice," and they don't really mean it, the plan cuts employees loose in a market of rapidly escalating health care costs. Those with limited funds will suffer as they are left to navigate for themselves in a market that is complex and confusing. The Internet, advocated by the proponents of "defined contributions" as a tool to educate consumers, is grossly overestimated in its usefulness. It's still a tool in its infancy, even for providers. The modern-day snake oil merchants, selling their expensive and sometimes marginally effective health care products and insurance, will retain their advantage.

Insurance companies are scrambling to design a variety of "defined-contribution" options for business. Once again we have vested interests, at least the insurance companies and employers, heading towards an option that places the interest of sick patients last. Many conservatives and physician groups, meanwhile, support close relatives of the "defined-contribution" approach: medical savings accounts, vouchers, and tax credits.

At some point we Americans will have to wake up. Perhaps our attachment to the mantra of "personal responsibility" and "the market" is so strong that we would actually support a solution under which some people can get PET scans, others leeches. Or maybe it's okay with us if low-income folks get a $10 991-minute phone card to talk to Dial-a-Nurse in Bangalore while wealthier Americans buy "concierge care" and have their own private physicians. Hopefully that kind of approach, or the reliance on bake-sale financing, will not be the "uniquely American" solution we choose. But while we're in health care "limbo," variations on the status quo will see us head in that very direction. And meanwhile the vested interests will continue to reap their profits since they hold the advantage in a game of "Survivor."

Maybe we need to reconsider our insistence on a "uniquely American" solution. Perhaps we need wake up, accept the obvious, put aside the myths, learn from the experience of other countries, and adopt a system based on "one risk pool" that gives every person in America affordable and accessible health care. Perhaps, as the famous Winston Churchill quote goes, we

Americans are destined to try every other system first, (including maybe even universal uninsurance), before we do the right thing.

Summary of Key Points

- America's health care financing system is unfair, illogical, costly, chaotic, confusing, absurd, and at times laughable.

- Our health care financing system is currently in danger of becoming even more complex and chaotic with some of the newer proposals (e.g., tax credits and vouchers) for "reducing the number of uninsured."

- We are headed towards a multi-tiered health care system in the U.S.—a system in which an increasing number of Americans (including many middle-class people) will be forced to play a game of "Survivor."

Only certain remedy for Rheumatism, Neuralgia, Headache, Piles, Sprains, and Bruises, Sores and Burns, Stiffness in the Joints: Salt Rheum, Felons, Frosted Hands, and Feet, Cramps in the Stomach, Palpitation and all kinds of Pains and Sores.

DISCOVERED AT LAST!!

Prof. DE GRATH'S "ELECTRIC OIL."

Greatest Cure in the World for Pains.

Chapter 14

Grassroots for Health Care for All: What Can Americans Do to Claim a Right to Health Care?

I have a fantasy. I see a huge football stadium full of people. Cheerleaders are leading the crowd: "Give me an H...." People in the stands turn over placards, one at a time. Finally, all the cards are up. They read "HEALTH CARE FOR ALL," and the crowd stomps and roars with approval.

I RECENTLY DID A personal mini-survey of the patients at my clinic. I asked why they thought the U.S., as opposed to all the other developed nations, did not guarantee health insurance to all its citizens. I got an interesting array of answers (see Chapter 5). Many replied, at least initially, that they didn't know why, or that "we couldn't afford it." But one 62-year-old woman asserted, "We need to unite, get together and demand universal coverage."

It's difficult to get large numbers of people interested in health care reform, let alone become activists. Discussions on health policy, if they go on for over a few minutes, more often than not get a glazed-eye response. Yet, without major popular support, without that stadium full of cheering people, movement towards any substantial reform—let alone a sweeping change such as national health insurance—will most likely remain a dream. Our political system makes this kind of fundamental change a daunting task. There are many other factors that also work against our efforts, including:

- The public's general lack of knowledge on the issue.

- Automatic prejudices, in the form of doubt-provoking sound bites, that have become a part of Americans' subconscious thinking. These attitudes have been created and reinforced by years of misinformation and myths.

- Politically and financially powerful corporate and medical interests (and their lobbyists and money), which are committed to stymie any efforts at change.

- A culture that generally believes in "market" solutions, individualism, and a "bootstrap" mentality, as opposed to health care as a basic human right.

- Habit. People are generally accepting of what they are accustomed to and fearful of change.

- For those Americans who are relatively well off, a sense of security in the status quo, a security that could somehow be threatened or lessened by change.

- Most people, especially middle-class insured people, have not had a personal bad experience with the system, at least up to now. They have been fairly well and have not had to use the system for any significant services.

- As such, most people are not "hurting enough" to get personally involved.

- Apathy. People, including physicians, are tied up in the hectic activities of their daily lives.

- Despite 9/11, Americans are not community-oriented people. Most Americans are more motivated to put the interests of the individual or the family first.

- The appearance that "something" is already being done. Incremental or piecemeal actions such as CHIP or "patient protection" acts may defuse some of the demand for action.

- Similarly, the high level of "lip service" to universal coverage with an array of complex and ineffectual proposals (but not national health insurance or Medicare for All).

This activity creates the impression that there is motion towards change.

- The whole movement towards universal coverage through national health insurance (NHI) lacks adequate financial support, as opposed to the well-heeled forces arrayed against NHI.

- The uninsured as a group are largely politically disenfranchised. They lack lobbyists or political clout.

- The failure of activists to agree upon a unified strategy or action plan to reach Health Care for All.

Facing these seemingly insurmountable obstacles, what steps can we take to create a groundswell of public support for Health Care for All?

Timing and the Changing Battlefield

IN NOVEMBER 2001, THE National Council on Health Care came out with an essay, "A Perfect Storm," by Joel Miller.[1] In this treatise, Miller postulates that there will soon be a convergence of the proper conditions to create an overwhelming public demand for universal coverage—akin to the weather conditions that made the "Perfect Storm" in the movie by that name. Other experts are also predicting that by 2003, economic conditions will force the U.S. to consider a major restructuring of its health care system. The principal converging factors: (a) a rapidly increasing number of uninsured and underinsured, (b) a marked rise in health insurance premiums and the cost of health care, (c) a worsening economy (which may be temporary, but will likely affect low-income people more), (d) a growing number of unemployed people, and (e) a demand for relief from employers. With all of the above conditions, state governments, which are already facing soaring expenditures for the Medicaid safety net, are likely to reach a state of fiscal panic.

Like the Taliban facing crisis conditions, the players on the health care battlefield could switch sides, even peaceably (see Chapter 12). Employers could demand relief and ask the government to take responsibility for insuring everyone. States will likely ask for a higher federal match for Medicaid. Harry and Louise could see the light, "get religion," realize there is a better way, and join the forces for universal coverage—maybe even national health insurance or an improved Medicare for All.

The corporate side will of course develop new strategies and permutations of the same old games to maximize the time they have to reap profits—in the same manner in which the pharmaceutical companies game the system to extend their patents. Universal coverage will continue to get lip service from all. There will be more "summits" to create the image that the elite care and are doing something to promote change. I personally won't believe they're serious about doing anything more than wringing the last dollar they can possibly squeeze out of the system until they put their money where their words are. Instead of seeing a $60 million ad campaign about the "bus from Canada," I'd like to see the drug companies, the insurance industry, and the AMA pool their resources on a $60 million publicity effort to persuade Americans to support national health insurance. It wouldn't be so impossible if business joined the bandwagon.

Timing is key. If the "Perfect Storm" should happen—and past forecasts of both weather and health care crises have been known to be fickle—then the grassroots support should be there to assure that the corporate guys can't pull off another shell game. The medical-industrial complex is not to be trusted. It can be held accountable if an informed and "hurting" public can be mobilized at the right time to fight for meaningful Health Care for All.

What do we Americans need to do to take advantage of the right moment, the magic hour when the stars are aligned just properly for health care reform? How can we be ready to "scramble" when the opportunity appears? Political winds can shift quickly, and openings for action can happen suddenly and disappear just as fast. We need to be prepared. If we're not ready, we could well wait another decade for the next opening. Realists would argue that, given the present administration in Washington, a reform as radical as national health insurance has about as much chance of passing as a snowball in hell. The Bush administration, if anything, has been promoting exactly the opposite: privatizing and/or dismembering Medicare—as well as Social Security. But 2004 is not far away. Already it appears there has been a prominent defector from the pro-privatization forces. In a campaign speech in Louisiana, Senator John Breaux (D-LA), who only a short while ago was promoting the privatization of Medicare, came out and said, "You ought to have health care as a basic right. Everybody in America should have health insurance and we should help people get it."[2] Politics acts in strange ways.

Groups, Old and New, Promoting Health Care for All

THE WALL STREET JOURNAL ran a front-page article on December 17, 2001, by Ron Winslow in which he talked about a rash of new organizations—he termed them "the sons of Jackson Hole"—that are working on solutions to our health care mess. Most of these didn't seem to be promoting Health Care for All. But a few new groups, like America's Health Together, are.

There are many other groups and/or coalitions that have been actively promoting universal coverage for years. Studying our health care system and the uninsured has been a major activity for some of these organizations, like the National Council on Health Care, which is comprised predominantly of major corporations. Education of the public has been a priority, although the degree of the public's knowledge so far has not been particularly impressive. Some foundations, like the Kaiser Family Foundation, have been cranking out useful information without endorsing a specific solution. Others, like the Commonwealth Fund, have financed numerous studies on the uninsured—and have also come up with specific proposals. One such plan came from Families USA, which joined with the Health Insurance Association of America (HIAA) to come up with the so-called "strange bedfellows" proposal for universal coverage.

On February 12, 2002, a day after President Bush's airing of his plans for health care, a group of 13 national organizations, led by the Robert Wood Johnson Foundation, came out with a new initiative that they named "CoveringTheUninsured."[3] They announced a $10 million television and print advertising campaign to publicize the plight of the uninsured. Part of their efforts are laudable, such as educating the American public about the obstacles faced by the uninsured or pointing out that 8 out of 10 uninsured Americans are in working families. Unfortunately, their initiative falls far short of what is needed. It may even signal a retreat from previous efforts that advocated for "universal coverage." In "seek[ing] solutions to the problem of the uninsured," they speak only of "reducing the number of the uninsured." They are clearly endorsing an "incremental" strategy, not universal coverage. One of its supporters rejected the single-payer approach as unaffordable. And only one of the sponsors, the Catholic Health Association, represented by Michael Collins, M.D., came out and specifically stated that *all Americans* should be afforded the justice of getting health care coverage, although John Sweeney, president of the AFL-CIO, did allude to "covering every American."

There is a general recognition that the American public has a woefully poor knowledge of what's happening in health care. The issues are difficult to explain because they are complex, confusing, and often politically charged. Physicians for a National Health Program (PNHP) has been striving over the past 15 years to educate primarily physicians but also others. PNHP uses hard data to show how America would benefit from national health insurance. PNHP researchers have also been documenting with studies how our system has been exploited and (literally) pillaged by investor-owned for-profit health care.

The public health community has been strongly supportive of Health Care for All. Medical groups such as the American Academy of Family Practice (AAFP) have laboriously developed proposals for universal coverage. The AAFP went so far as to propose truly universal coverage (everybody in) for primary care and prevention, with a publicly administered system that abolishes the employer link and has tax-based financing.

The ACP-ASIM (the internal medicine specialists) actually spent a million dollars to buy ads promoting universal coverage. And in April 2002, they came out with a stepwise (over seven years) proposal that would provide health insurance coverage for every American. Their proposal is based on the expansion of Medicaid and CHIP plus premium support, so it fails to address the issue of affordability and leaves our fragmented, overly complex, and wasteful system intact. At least they're sincere in their efforts. A few professional groups, like the American Nurses Association (ANA) and the American Medical Students Association (AMSA), have been solid national health insurance supporters for years.

The Community-Based Efforts

IN ADDITION TO THE professional groups that are pushing for health care reform and universal coverage, there are many community-based groups that are fighting for Health Care for All at the state level. California has already had two ballot initiatives that would have mandated single-payer universal coverage for the state. Both failed, as did a similar ballot initiative in Massachusetts in 2000. The latter lost by 52 percent to 48 percent, thanks to a last-minute $6 million advertising blitz from the insurance companies. State-based groups in over 20 states have been pressing for universal coverage. In some states, like Maine, where there has been effective campaign finance reform, the approach has been through legislative action. Both of Maine's legislative chambers actually passed a single-payer bill in 2001. But they had to amend their bill because the Governor threatened to veto it. A more developed proposal was to come back in 2002, but has been "put on hold."

In November 2001, voters in Portland, Maine, passed a non-binding referendum endorsing single-payer universal coverage despite being vastly outspent by the opposition. Anthem Blue Shield, a for-profit insurer (and the largest insurer in Maine), spent nearly $400,000 on advertising in the last two weeks before the vote in an attempt to convince the voters to reject the referendum. The supporters of single-payer universal coverage only had about $15,000 to spend, but they won. Their victory inspired speculation that the time was propitious for a new national debate on health care.[4] In other states, like Oregon and Washington, there are current efforts to win universal coverage through ballot or legislative initiatives.

Recently, the Health Resources Service Administration (HRSA), part of HHS, gave about a million dollars to each of 20 states to study the problems of the uninsured in their respective states and to come up with some options for decreasing the numbers of the uninsured. The grants' stated purpose was actually to promote getting insurance coverage for "all," but the "all" got diluted out in practice. However, at least in Idaho, and I'm sure in other states as well, the grant served the purpose of helping to educate health care leaders and legislators (and the public, though to a much lesser degree) on the issues surrounding the uninsured. Idaho's legislators, for example, were surprised to learn that 80 percent of the uninsured were people in working families. And useful studies came out of the HRSA grants, like the cost analyses of single-payer universal coverage that were done in Vermont and California. Both showed that the single-payer approach would not only cover everyone, but also save five percent overall.

At the Congressional level, there has been some simmering activity to try to lay the groundwork for Health Care for All—and promise of some real action in the near future. So far, there has been little current support for broad proposals, like Bill Clinton's ill-fated "Managed Competition for All" plan or Jim McDermott's (D-WA) HR 1200. The latter had at one point garnered 140 cosponsors for single-payer universal coverage. But there has been talk of bills to facilitate state-by-state single-payer efforts as well as to provide waivers so the federal programs can be included in a state's single-payer plan. On May 1, 2001, progressive representatives held a Congressional hearing in which a standing ovation was given for a sweeping single-payer proposal. And Representative John Conyers (D-MI) is about to introduce a new single-payer bill.

Meanwhile, there has been a movement to gain support for universal coverage through House Concurrent Resolution

(HCR) 99. This resolution, also called the "Health Care Access Resolution," lists and endorses all the positive features of Health Care for All, but avoids mentioning any specific approach. Its supporters, which include many activist organizations, seem to be trying to stay on politically safe ground so they can garner more general support for universal coverage itself. It's unclear if the proponents of HCR 99 are laying the groundwork to build general support for what will become national health insurance. Yet it's hard to imagine that the principles outlined in the resolution, if implemented, could be anything but a national health insurance solution. Some of the backers of HCR 99, however, may have given up on a truly comprehensive solution, and may be seeking "the best they can get" for the American people. An April 30, 2002, panel discussion of HCR 99 can be viewed on <www.kff.org>, the website of the Kaiser Family Foundation.

On the Internet, there are now a host of websites that disseminate useful information about our health care system and its problems, including <www.pnhp.org>, <www.cmwf.org>, <www.kff.org>, and <www.everybodyinnobodyout.org>, to mention but a few.

More Talk, Less Progress?

DESPITE ALL THE EFFORTS of these groups to raise America's consciousness of our problems with health care, there continues to be a very high level of cluelessness at all levels, from the general public to our leaders, and even health care professionals. There also is a worrisome level of disagreement among activist groups about strategy. Some would describe the split as one between pragmatists and idealists. Only two or three years ago, there seemed to be some strong consensus for a single-payer solution, like an improved Medicare for All. But, perhaps out of frustration or impatience—or pragmatism—many former single-payer advocates, like UHCAN (Universal Health Coverage for America Network), modified their demand for national health insurance. Some past supporters of the single-payer approach have gone so far as to assert, "If you insist on holding out for single payer, you'll get nothing!" In a September 27, 2001, MSNBC editorial, University of Pennsylvania bioethicist Art Caplan took that position (see Chapter 16).

Some former single-payer supporters have come to the conclusion that the American people have suffered enough and it's better to do something incremental rather than hold out for the elusive "big enchilada" or "brass ring." In a similar struggle of political pragmatism versus idealism, the 2002 Maryland universal coverage initiative changed course and dropped its single-payer orientation. That initiative had garnered support from an amazing array of organizations from all around Maryland, but the organizers perceived that the initiative would fail if it didn't embrace a "pluralistic" approach instead of single payer. So, arguing that something is better than nothing, they compromised and took a more incremental approach. The end result (and many uninsured people) will also be compromised if the initiative passes.

In the everyday real world of health care, all of us who work with health get involved with so-called "incremental" actions. We try to qualify people for Medicaid. We lobby so that SCHIP funding will not be cut. We volunteer at free clinics. We fight to get support for Critical Access Hospitals. Some health care activists argue for doing absolutely nothing—so that the whole system will implode sooner. But being the compassionate people we are, the nihilist ("tough love") approach is hard to accept when we see so much injustice and need. How can we stand by and do nothing tangible? The collective mission of grassroots activists should be to remind each other (in the words of Darth Vader) to "keep our eye on the leader"—to maintain the vision. The ultimate goal ("leader") is universal coverage that is affordable, comprehensive, and equitable.

Meanwhile, we fight the daily skirmishes—because we have to—while keeping our eye on the prize. It is unfortunate that activist groups cannot be more united in their strategies and messages. As time passes, however, the level of consciousness should increase. When that rising level of consciousness meets an escalating level of "public pain," the time will be ripe for meaningful reform—assuming a few more stars, like the political will, are lined up correctly. We should hold steady on our goal of national health insurance, but it may well require a "next best step" strategy, like stepwise expansion of Medicare or a state-by-state approach to get the process rolling.

What Specific Action Steps Will It Take to Motivate Grassroots America?

As HAS BEEN BRIEFLY outlined above, an impressive amount of groundwork has already been done at many levels to create an infrastructure that can be used to promote Health Care for All in America. But because the issue is so complex and confusing, it's relatively easy for the well-heeled opponents of meaningful health care reform to derail progress towards a solution such as national health insurance. All they need to do to obstruct change is create doubt among the public and our political leaders. To effect their negative objectives, they have huge financial resources. And they have access to the politicians, access they have facilitated through campaign contributions.

Given the power of the medical-industrial complex, what can be done, what specific action steps can activists take to win over the hearts and souls of grassroots America? How can we get ordinary Americans to support Health Care for All? Part of the answer must come from addressing the problem areas outlined at the beginning of this chapter. In brief, some likely (and practical) steps would be:

- Develop, with the help of publicists, a series of simple, to the point, targeted messages[5] to change how people respond to Health Care for All and to counter the gut-level sound bites that stop the conversation. We are selling a good product. The opposition is selling "snake oil." We need to get our message out effectively and often.

- The specific countermessages we need to develop, and deliver with a positive twist, should address "the government," rationing, choice, affordability, and "the unknown," including "what's it going to cost me," health care in other countries, and "socialized medicine." It needs to be stressed that the delivery system will remain predominantly private, as it is now.

- Develop a plan to get maximum media exposure through a variety of strategies that we can afford, and get the timing correct. The opposition has megabucks, knows how to use proper timing, and can afford to buy space on prime time TV, not just at 3 a.m. Again, use professional help, develop a series of themes that seem hopeful, experiment, change course if they don't seem to be working, and concentrate efforts on those approaches that work.

- Prepare a series of position fliers that are brief, simple, easy to understand, and can be used to counter the misinformation and myths from the opposition. Give these materials wide circulation and try to be sure they are used in a timely manner, when an issue has the spotlight.

- Take advantage of every opportunity to rebut regressive proposals from the medical-industrial establishment— and in a timely manner. Call-in radio, op-eds, letters to the editor, input at forums. A coordinated information bulletin board with alerts to activists and a method to stimulate specific action at the right moment so that it gets the most media exposure. We have the means for communication: the Internet. But we need some group or groups to coordinate the effort, to act as "command headquarters."

- Have a "quick-response" team, linked by the Internet, that can respond quickly to opportunities to get the message out and counter the other side's actions.

- Seek foundation support to get our message out, to educate the public.

- Recruit some famous people to be visible and outspoken in support of the cause. Win Harry and Louise to our side, "the better way."

- Target politicians and community leaders at every level to hear our message. There are potentially millions of ad-hoc lobbyists (activists and short-changed patients) whose passion can make more of an impression than the calculated retorts from paid lobbyists.

- Be sure our message gets out to all the groups and "summits" that are thinking about universal coverage. If we are excluded, find ways to be sure our message is heard—from carefully targeting key people with personally presented information to (if necessary) public demonstrations or even civil disobedience.[6]

- Work together so that we coordinate the battle and target our efforts to where they will be most effective. There may be disagreements on strategies among different activist groups, but we should all strive to agree on the ultimate goal.

- Develop a nationwide network of activists and community people who are willing to be (a) local leaders and (b) foot soldiers for the cause.

- Convince the opposition to join us (see Chapter 12). Target specific groups that could be recruited to be allies in the cause: small business, human rights groups, church groups, unions, big business, sympathetic professional societies (perhaps in that order). Have a coordinated campaign to do the recruitment, probably on a state-by-state level.

- Convince state legislators that Health Care for All can save their states money by providing a method to limit Medicaid expenditures.

- Continue to work on state-level efforts, such as initiatives and legislation, because they help bring attention to the cause, make the issue visible at the local level, and educate the public. They may even represent our "best chance" as a step to reach national health insurance—or an end in itself if America espouses a federalist (state-by-state) approach. We should continue to encourage out-of-state activists to help bolster a state's cause.

- Appeal to a sense of community. "We're all in this together." The same argument should be made for affordability. We pay more for the uninsured in the long run because they delay needed care, come in sicker, and require more expensive treatment that we all, as a society, wind up paying for.

What I've outlined above looks challenging. It looks like a political campaign. And it is. Flexibility and the ability to have a rapid response will be key elements to assure success. We cannot ignore grassroots support even if a top-down effort at universal coverage, like a ballot initiative or legislation, succeeds. Experience teaches us that we must have the grassroots with us because the corporate interests have managed to reverse some short-lived victories in the past (e.g., Massachusetts and Washington).

What we're lacking is effective and coordinated leadership— and money. The vested interests have an abundance of cash, but we have the passion and a just cause. However, if we want to be effective, we will need to work together and pool our resources, both human and financial. Unlike the pharmaceutical or insurance industries, we can't drop a few million dollars at a moment's notice to create a "front" organization or finance a publicity campaign.

We need to be wary of the corporate "moles" who sponsor sweet-sounding "summits" that go nowhere. Separating out the corporate infiltrators, the rest of us activists need to collaborate despite philosophical disagreements because it's an uphill battle. America remains clueless. We argue over the meaning of incremental, sometimes trying to distinguish such terms as "incremental" and "sequential" from "piecemeal." But we can agree to disagree, and work together effectively, if we all keep our attention on the prize: comprehensive and affordable health care for everyone in America, as with national health insurance or an improved Medicare for All. The ultimate "interest" we are pursuing is the best interest of every patient—and that's all of us. And, after all (as discussed below in Chapter 18), Health Care for All is an "incremental" step in itself; what we're really after is Good Health for All. On the way there, however, it would sure be encouraging to hear a roar from the stadium. "Give me an H!"

Summary of Key Points

- The system is stacked against the grassroots activists and the American people, but time is on their side.

- An increasing number of groups are pressing for meaningful change through a variety of mechanisms, including ballot initiatives and legislative action.

- There has been a worrisome recent trend to shift the goal away from universal coverage to "reducing the number of the uninsured."

- It will be a challenge involving widespread community efforts to win Health Care for All.

Chapter 15

National Health Insurance
or Medicare for All:
A Reality in Our Lifetime?

*There's an anecdote that relates what happened to a
health care activist who toiled for many years for the
cause of universal coverage. When she died, she went to
heaven where she met God at the pearly gates. "God,"
she asked, "will there ever be universal coverage for
health care in America?" God pondered the question for
a minute and then replied, "Yes, indeed, but not in my lifetime."*

AT THE BEGINNING OF the 21st century, there seems to be
a sense of frustration or even hopelessness over the prospect of
ever getting to universal coverage. Especially distant is the hope
for a truly seamless system that would include *everybody*, such as
an improved Medicare for All. Yet, I somehow cannot put out of
my mind—perhaps I am paranoid—that this aura of impossibility
has been created and kept alive by the vested interests of the
medical-industrial complex, the merchants of misinformation
and myth.

Speaking to a special Congressional hearing, Marcia Angell,
the former editor-in-chief of the *New England Journal of
Medicine*, strongly decried as a myth the idea that America could
not reach universal coverage using a single-payer system (see
Chapter 1, Myth #13). Of course, there is a whole litany of
myths about American health care (again, see Chapter 1) including, "We can get to universal coverage through an incremental
approach."

The increased interest in universal coverage that began to be evident in the late '90s was expressed in a September 6, 1999, *New York Times* editorial. It called attention to "...this country's grievous failure to provide coverage for nearly one-sixth of its population.... The problem remains a vivid and embarrassing rebuke to American democracy." A later editorial from the same newspaper, published September 24, 2000, queried, "...If this moment—a moment of unprecedented economic prosperity and looming budget surpluses—is the wrong one for an aggressive move towards universal health insurance, when will it be right?" Although the projected budget surpluses are now ancient history, the need for universal coverage has not gone away. It's possible that the switch to "looming budget deficits" could inspire and accomplish what the surpluses could not.

It's Become Fashionable to Talk About Universal Coverage

SINCE THE LATE '90s—perhaps enough time had passed since the Clinton health plan collapsed—there has been a flurry of proposals to cover the uninsured. Many medical societies have come up with plans, as have foundations and institutes, such as the Commonwealth Fund and the Economic and Social Research Institute.[1] And there have been a variety of "summits" convened to talk about the issue.

However, the gist of most of the new proposals has not really been "universal," despite the rhetoric. Simple, comprehensive, and understandable proposals, such as the 2001 call for "Medicare for All" from the Economic Policy Institute,[2] have been in the minority. There even seems to be a more recent trend to replace the term "universal coverage" with "reducing the number of uninsured." Such is the case with the $10 million advertising campaign initiated in February 2002 by a new coalition of 13 organizations called "Covering the Uninsured."[3] Single-payer, "one risk pool," and Medicare for All advocates seem to have been purposefully excluded, even uninvited, from national "summits" on universal coverage. Nancy Dickey, the former president of the American Medical Association (AMA), while speaking at a meeting of the American Public Health Association, seemed to indicate there wasn't even a place at the table for single-payer advocates.

My untrusting side makes me wonder if the chief sponsors of the "summits" on universal coverage—the AMA and the pharmaceutical industry—may have had a hidden agenda in mind when they excluded single-payer advocates from their deliberations. After all, the AMA has been steadfastly against solutions like an improved Medicare for All. Their official, and oft repeated, position is that, "Single-payer systems are not in the best interests of the public, physicians or the health care of this nation and should be strenuously resisted." The AMA has managed to derail every universal coverage proposal over the past nine decades. Somehow, despite their strong opposition, Medicare, the limited single-payer plan for Americans 65 years old and over, got through in 1965.

As for the pharmaceutical industry, a national health insurance plan could be a disaster for their bottom line—or so they think, though it might not be so bad for them. It could mean an end to their ability to exploit the market so as to assure the highest price for their products. Why should the vested interests support real change when they can do piecemeal approaches that basically keep the status quo? Minor modifications that only tweak the system allow them to keep their primacy in the market and their profits. To give the appearance of being good guys, they can talk about universal coverage and then dismiss it as being unrealistic.

So these powers that be (a.k.a., "the Evil Empire" of the health care industry) have created the myth that America cannot, and will not, accept Medicare for All, or the equivalent. Who controls the media? Who has the ear of politicians? Who has the money to drop a few million dollars on an advertising campaign to derail an effort at universal coverage or to sink a proposal to put meaningful pharmaceutical benefits into Medicare?

Even the executive director at my community health center, though an advocate for universal coverage, frequently expresses his skepticism. "Do you really think we'll have universal coverage anytime soon? In our lifetimes?" he asks. And a well-meaning caller to the Eugene, OR, NPR affiliate, where I participated in a talk show, asked about a compromise quasi-universal proposal, insuring all kids progressively from birth, while making the assumption that a quicker process to cover everyone was politically impossible.

Some of the proposals for so-called "universal coverage," such as the Commonwealth Fund's idea, which falls short of really being universal, remind me of what happened when the last great debate on universal coverage took place in 1993–94. Great minds in Washington argued over whether 95 percent or 92 percent coverage satisfied the criterion for universal. I'm convinced that if we adopt something like the Commonwealth Fund's proposal, we will only perpetuate the wastefulness and administrative complexity of the current system. And we will continue to exclude many of the patients whom I (and others who take care of the uninsured) see personally. Those are the people who fall between the cracks because of their incomes and/or eligibility criteria.

It reminds me of a young man in Oregon who related how he earned just a few dollars too much to qualify for the Oregon Health Plan, or the single mom from Eugene who was careful not to earn too much money so her children could continue to qualify for Medicaid. Including everybody automatically would be so simple, so fair, and save so much on administrative costs, that one would think it would be a no-brainer. But such inclusiveness would limit how the vested interests could game the system. Those interests, the very same interests that a Commonwealth Fund-type proposal would serve, would prefer to shift all high-risk patients to government-paid programs. The private sector would retain the low-risk people (the well)—i.e., the profitable segment of our population.

Why Don't the People Who Know Better Do Something?

WHAT IS MOST DISAPPOINTING to me is the lack of support—or is it resignation?—from people who deal on a daily basis with the uninsured. There is a wide gap between the rhetoric and action.

The U.S. Public Health Service (PHS) and the Health Resources Service Administration (HRSA) have a prominent campaign to reduce health disparities to zero. A major goal of the PHS' effort called *Healthy People 2010* is that all Americans will have health insurance coverage by that date (it was also an objective for *Healthy People 2000*). Since having health insurance would without doubt be the single most effective measure to reduce racial disparities in health care and improve health status, why do we see so little action from the people in community health centers and the PHS community in support of a solution like national health insurance?

They can't possibly fail to appreciate the lower rates of insurance coverage in minority groups. The Census Bureau figures for 1999 show uninsurance rates of 33.5 percent for Hispanics and 22 percent for blacks, compared to 11 percent for non-Hispanic whites. In March 2002, the Commonwealth Fund released a study assessing health care quality and minority Americans.[4] Their conclusion: "Perhaps most fundamental to ensuring quality medical care for minority Americans is the availability of affordable, comprehensive health insurance."

Are HRSA and the PHS, not to mention the National Association of Community Health Centers (NACHC), afraid to speak up because they are (to a greater or lesser degree) dependent upon an administration that does not officially support such a solution? Are they playing politics so they can be assured that they will continue to have their portion of the health care pie in our fragmented system? Or are they simply too tied up in their daily work, with endless hours spent in pursuit of grants? They chase grants to support one part of the puzzle, while they're trying to nail down a sub-program to tie together with some other program (both of which will expire in a year or two). All of these efforts are directed toward meeting the needs of their uninsured or inadequately insured patients. It would be great if all these efforts could go to benefit the patients in need instead of seeking ways to get through wasteful and often counterproductive administrative mazes.

There is also a general assumption, perhaps reinforced by the stand of the AMA, that physicians in general are opposed to the single-payer type solution. But a national study of academic physicians, residents and medical students published in the *New England Journal of Medicine* in 1999 revealed that 57 percent of the respondents felt the single-payer option "would offer the best care to the greatest number of people."[5] A 2001 survey of Massachusetts physicians (in a state where a 2000 ballot initiative for universal coverage lost by only a four percent margin) revealed that 66 percent of the physicians felt single payer was the preferred option for reform. However, only 51 percent thought that most physicians they knew supported it.

The Naysayers' Logic

OPPOSITION TO A TYPE of solution like national health insurance or an improved "Medicare for All" comes from people who object to giving government such a large role. They fail to realize that government is already footing the lion's share of our spending for health care. If we factor in the costs of Medicare, Medicaid, the Veterans Administration, the National Institutes of Health, the Defense Department, public hospitals, health departments, community and rural health centers, the tax subsidy to employer-supplied health insurance, the spending of state and local governments on premiums, and workmen's compensation, "government" spending already accounts for over 60 percent of all health care spending in the U.S.[6] Private employers contribute less than 20 percent to the overall costs, with individual spending making up the rest.

The naysayers say they don't like making health care "an entitlement" or a right. We as a nation, supposedly being more attuned to individualism, have not yet embraced the concept of health care as a human right—as has every other industrialized democracy. The detractors of national health insurance or "Medicare for All" prefer giving more prominence to the concept of "personal responsibility." Perhaps for them, responsibly paying your taxes, which pay for Medicare, doesn't count. However, it seems it's the rich folks and corporate America, like Enron, that are best at finding ways to avoid paying taxes.

Analyzed properly, the "personal responsibility" gig is an excuse to "blame the victims." If a person has paid his taxes, he/she has in essence paid a premium for a health insurance plan called Medicare. The fiscal responsibility has been met. And this concept is applicable whether it's Medicare for people over 65 or Medicare for All. That leaves the "personal responsibility" mantra as a ploy to (a) justify co-pays or (b) punish the poor, who often can't afford the co-pays and thus delay care.

The objections to national health insurance or Medicare for All are partly philosophical but largely economic. Of course, it's ironic that the AMA should be so anti-Medicare. Although recent high-handed HCFA (now CMS) tactics have made the doctors angry, Medicare made the doctors rich—despite the AMA's original opposition to the program.

How about looking at this issue from the point of view that *really* counts, the interests of the American people? What are the real worries that we should be concerned about if we were to have a solution like an "improved Medicare for All?" A "single risk pool" with all 280 million Americans in, and nobody out. From the patients' (as well as the providers') viewpoints, the concerns would be:

- The level of bureaucracy. The degree of regulation needs to be appropriate to assure accountability but not be overpowering. Vast simplification, including everybody-in eligibility and a well-understood (and comprehensive) benefit package, should facilitate the process of designing a user-friendly system that minimizes bureaucracy. A system that is more transparent will also lessen the need for bureaucracy. And there must be built-in mechanisms to allow easy public input into the system. The type of bureaucracy embodied in today's Medicare is not acceptable and will require improvement.

- Flexibility. Build into the design a degree of local control and administration so that individual needs can be appropriately addressed. The system design must include an ability to be responsive to changing needs, including ways to encourage and enhance research, training, and excellence in health care.

- The winds of politics. As with the current situation, politics can affect the whole system—especially financing. That's why the system should have a separate trust fund, insulated from being raided to serve other needs.

- Choice and access. Likely not real worries. Choice should be much improved, since a patient could have full choice of any provider, unlike the current system. As for access, it would also be greatly improved overall, although there could be some local variations in access when the financing mechanism changes.

- Inefficiency and corruption/fraud. These are the standard conservative's worries about anything that is "government-run." Health care in America is already so inefficient (with Medicare being perhaps the most financially efficient, even in its current state, see Chapter 1, Myth #4) that this aspect could only be made better with national health insurance or an improved Medicare for All. As for fraud, a transparent system with fewer complexities can only serve to diminish fraud (see Chapter 2). And as to the fear about being "government-run," the delivery system would remain predominantly private, as it is today.

- "Rationing" of services. A fear that with budget shortfalls there could be a compromise in the benefit package. Decisions on benefits belong in a public forum, and a mechanism to provide public input into the decision-making process must be built into any reforms.

The myth of "Why we can't have national health insurance, or Medicare for All," builds upon many other myths about America's health care system. The politically based and economically motivated rhetoric has been designed to subvert any real change. "Americans want more choice, Medicare is going broke, we don't want big government, we don't want more taxes." And even a call for "compassion" (versus justice). Plant doubt. Play on people's fears.

Is it possible, in the spirit of American free enterprise exemplified by Enron, HCA/Columbia, WorldCom, and the pharmaceutical giants who pay off smaller companies *not* to produce generics, that the major economic powers within the health industry got together and decided to systematically exclude solutions like national health insurance? Savvy as they are on health care, it's hard to believe that the economic powers of our health care industry do not realize, deep in their hearts, that a single-payer type of universal coverage, with "one risk pool," is what America needs. A parallel situation might be that of the tobacco industry, which for years denied that smoking caused cancer—even though they knew all along that it did. Like the tobacco industry, the health care industry knows that it is to their own economic interests to milk the system for as long as they can. And that's why a person like Tom Scully, the Administrator of CMS, can assert with a straight face, at a National Health Policy Conference in 2002, that even doing limited fixes to Medicare and Medicaid will take 10 to 25 years.

After all, our current health care system isn't wasteful to the insurance industry, the pharmaceutical companies, the for-profit HMOs and hospitals, and some of the more lucrative parts of the medical profession. They can maintain the standard litany of myths while they continue to oppose meaningful reforms, such as national health insurance or a real pharmaceutical benefit within Medicare. It may take a cataclysmic event, or maybe a combination of really adverse economic conditions as Joel Miller describes in his essay "The Perfect Storm,"[7] to shake us up. Maybe then we'll see Health Care for All or even a single-payer type solution like national health insurance.

Summary of Key Points

- There may be a conspiracy of the "vested interests" to keep single-payer national health insurance off the table.

- An improved and expanded Medicare for All offers a good starting framework and/or conceptual model for an American system of universal coverage.

- Without affordable, comprehensive health insurance for everyone, the goal of "zero disparities" for minority health care will not be realized.

- "Government" already finances about 60 percent of all health care costs in the U.S. Private employers contribute less than 20 percent.

- A litany of myths from the "vested interests" helps to block universal coverage and maintain the status quo.

- It may take a combination of cataclysmic events to act as a stimulus for real change.

Chapter 16

"Single Payer Will Not Fly": A Response[1]

"Single payer will not fly. Period. I favor it but it has no chance, none, nada, zero with Bush in and the Republicans in Congress.... My view is: forget about doing best. It is time to do better. Let's get something. Fifty years of waiting for a national health system has left tens of millions with nothing...."

— Arthur Caplan, Ph.D., director of the Center for Bioethics at the University of Pennsylvania, October 2001, in an e-mail to Ida Hellander, M.D., executive director of Physicians for a National Health Program

IS NATIONAL HEALTH INSURANCE, or "single-payer" reform a pipe dream in America? Should Americans be settling for something less? Often this "best" option, "best" at least from the viewpoint of the American people, is abruptly dismissed with a snicker and a curt, "Forget it, it's politically impossible." I had to face that attitude recently when I was discussing a single-payer approach as one of the options for increasing coverage in Idaho. And I had to admit that—given the complexity of the whole issue and the level of understanding, as well as the philosophical bias of Idaho's politicians—it would be a hard sell. Idaho has the most Republican (89 percent) legislature in America.

The myth that single payer is impossible in America has been propagated by special interests in order to cut off any discussion of single payer as an option (see Chapter 15). When a group of health care organizations put out their "Joint Statement" on universal coverage in 1999, they specifically specified that any solution had to be "pluralistic," thus automatically excluding the single-payer approach while mandating a "poison pill" that makes simplification of our fragmented system nearly impossible. Single-payer advocates were not even allowed at the discussion.

Does "Incremental" Have a Chance?

THE MYTH ASIDE, WILL a "something" solution cure our wasteful and badly fragmented health care system? Can we scrape together enough crumbs so that, even if we don't have the whole cake, the health care needs of the American people will be satisfied? I think these questions bring us back to the overall feasibility of "incremental" changes (see Chapter 1, Myth #12, for more discussion). Can "incremental" work? There's no doubt that incremental changes, though at best only marginally effective, are politically feasible. But our recent experiments with a series of incremental proposals have only seemed to buy time for the special interests, time during which the plight of the American people, and their access to health care, has only gotten worse. Some groups of Americans have been included (e.g., as with CHIP) while other groups (e.g., those millions with ever-increasing deductibles and co-pays) have been experiencing increased difficulty in accessing care.

We have experimented with (and continue to toy with) medical savings accounts, Medicare+Choice (which, ironically, has often meant less choice), Medicaid managed care, the CHIP program, guaranteed issue insurance, small group insurance purchasing, catastrophic funds, and a variety of Medicaid expansions. The most current proposals *du jour* are now tax credits and "defined contributions." And soon we will be hearing about "personal health accounts." With the possible exception of the managed-care approaches, all of these incremental efforts have zero potential for changing a system that is broken. In fact, they fragment the system even more by making it even more complicated and administratively wasteful.

As for the managed-care approaches, such as Medicare+ Choice, they have often only served to increase overall cost—the opposite of their intended goal. Moreover, they have led to an accentuation of the problem of risk avoidance or "cherry picking," a problem which only a "single risk pool," or national health insurance, can solve. As for one of today's "poster child" solutions—refundable tax credits, the complexity of this proposal is so extreme that it is difficult to believe that serious thinkers can even realistically consider the option. Perhaps it would serve the interests of single-payer proponents to actually have a go at refundable tax credits. The resulting implosion of the financing system, which is headed towards meltdown anyway, would require a more radical fix, like national health insurance.

How About Affordability for the Patient?

INCREASINGLY, WE NEED TO deal with the question of affordability. And that question has two sides, one of which we have so far neglected to address as a nation. We have given attention to and worried about affordability from the viewpoint of our national and state budgets. And politicians have been sensitive to the increasing health insurance cost burden on business and industry. But in comparison to the attention given to costs for government and industry, almost no attention has been devoted to the cost of health care borne by the patient or consumer. Instead, the patient has been increasingly squeezed with a spiral of higher deductibles and co-payments. And people who have been sick are penalized even more, especially if they have an awful "pre-existing condition," with astronomical prices for health insurance, if it's even available. The "incremental" approaches have done nothing to improve this situation. Nor do such approaches have the potential to deal with these kinds of problems.

Admittedly, I am biased by the patients I see on a daily basis at my community health center—over half of whom are uninsured. When I consider my low-income patients, the various piecemeal proposals—medical savings accounts, tax credits, and small group arrangements to buy bare-bones coverage—seem like pipe dreams as opposed to single payer. It totally depends on the angle from which one looks at what needs to be done. From the politicians' angle, influenced by the best information and biases that money can buy and a philosophy that holds on to the impossible dream that "the market" can solve our health care woes, single-payer national health insurance seems a political impossibility. Yet, to the American people (all of us who are patients/consumers, and especially those of us who are squeezed by health care costs or simply unable to afford health care at all), single-payer national health insurance is probably the *only* solution that will work. Other solutions, the incremental type, not only will continue to perpetuate an increasingly complex and wasteful system, but also will create new cracks in our already profusely leaking series of safety nets. If the American public really understood what the trade-offs were, they—instead of corporate America—could apply pressure to our politicians that would make national health insurance a political reality instead of a political pariah.

Consistent with our head-in-the-sand approach to international matters in general, we have ignored or purposively degraded through disinformation campaigns the experiences of other countries (e.g., Canada). No foreign health care system is perfect, but the developed countries do cover everybody, and they do spend a fraction of what we spend—while we fail to cover over 40 million Americans and expose even more to financial ruin should they be so unlucky as to incur a serious illness or injury.

The question remains, can we make the situation "better" without a "single risk pool" or without universal coverage? Even a state-by-state strategy or the expansion of Medicare to an entire age group, such as every child or everyone 55–64 years old, could serve as a starting point. But without a single-payer approach, we will just be playing the poke-the-balloon game, where pushing a finger in one spot just creates a blip on the other side.

"Best" vs. "Better": In Search of Value for Our Money

WE COULD ACCOMPLISH SOME changes, though I'm not sure it would meet the definition of "better," by throwing more money at the system. The simplest approach would be to increase eligibility for Medicaid or CHIP, as many states have already done and as some national schemes propose (including the ACP-ASIM proposal for universal coverage), thus increasing the enrollment of low-income people in these plans. But Medicaid is very unpopular among politicians in most states and carries the stigma of "welfare." And states are now frantically trying to limit their Medicaid spending. Moreover, access to providers is limited because of its low reimbursement.

The fiscal implications would be significant, but if it's only a question of money, theoretically we could greatly expand Medicaid to cover, say, everyone up to 300 percent of the federal poverty level. Or we could simply buy commercial health insurance for every American, as the tax credit or rebate proposal tries to do, or as in Arthur Caplan's voucher proposal. That approach, however, wouldn't solve the problem for high-risk individuals or families, unless we were also willing to pick up their $1000-a-month-with-$5000-deductible premiums. The sky's the limit if we want to use our imagination and bankroll anything.

However, I think there's some political—and practical and ethical—advantage in getting some value for what we spend. And that value depends very much on having a cohesive financing system that can share the risk, set priorities, use scientific and information-based health care modalities (including prevention), and have some vision for what America needs. Our fragmented system does virtually none of the above. Nor does our system give a proper place to prevention (see the following chapter) in addressing the issue of affordability.

It appears likely that, at least for the immediate future, we will continue on the piecemeal track. Many, including myself, will work on proposals to make access "better," knowing that "better" is a slippery slope, perhaps leading nowhere. In time, possibly sooner rather than later, the stars will align to make the time right for national health insurance—likely *de facto* single payer but with some limited role for our insurance industry. The events of September 11 may have helped to bring into play some of the necessary change elements, such as a sense of community and some decrease in our disdain for government. But it will take a critical mass of hurting Americans—and a better public understanding of a complex issue—to create the grassroots groundswell that will make national health insurance politically acceptable.

Meanwhile, personally I'll continue striving for "best"— national health insurance with "one risk pool"—because that's what my patients deserve.

Summary of Key Points

- Incremental changes can only be minimally effective in attaining meaningful health care reform.

- We will not have health care justice or affordability unless we include every person in America in "one risk pool," simplify the system, and reduce administrative costs—all impossible with the kinds of incremental approaches being proposed.

- Unless we choose the "best" solution—as opposed to piecemeal approaches—most of my patients will continue to do without needed health care.

Chapter 17

Needed for Affordable and Effective Health Care Reform in America: A Paradigm Shift for Prevention

The speaker at the closing day general session of the annual meeting of the American College of Preventive Medicine was expounding about how exercise as a routine way of life had not yet become mainstream in America. The day before, I had locked my bicycle to a bench across from the entrance to the five-star hotel in New Orleans where the meeting was being held. Hotel people snipped a cable lock and disassembled the bench so they could remove the bike, which they undoubtedly considered unworthy of gracing the front of their upscale hotel. When the speaker finished, I related—to the delight of the audience—the bike story to illustrate that America still has a long way to go to make exercise an accepted part of our daily lives. It's probably some consolation to remember that a mere 25 years ago, meetings of the College took place in smoke-filled rooms. Change can happen.

AFFORDABILITY IS A CRITICAL part of the solution to making "Health Care for All" possible. And prevention—*real* prevention—has a key role (along with administrative savings) in making "Health Care for All" affordable. Although there is some controversy over how much some clinical preventive measures actually save overall, the more basic prevention activities, such as immunizations and prenatal care, have been clearly demonstrated to save money for our society as a whole. For example, it

222

is generally agreed that for every dollar we spend on prenatal care, we save $7 in the long run. And a smoking cost study released in April 2002 by the Centers for Disease Control and Prevention (CDC)[1] calculated how much money our society could save by reducing the use of tobacco products. The study put the nation's total cost of smoking at $157.7 billion a year, or $7 for every pack smoked, about evenly split between smoking-related medical costs and lost job productivity. Dealing with our nation's epidemic of obesity probably offers even greater possibilities for overall cost savings (see below).

The traditional medical care approach to assuring good health has its limits. New technologies have opened up a myriad of wonderful new possibilities for health care. And the future will undoubtedly see an increasing number of therapeutic advances capable of both improving and extending our lives—assuming we're fortunate enough to have access to them. But economic, environmental, societal, public health, and lifestyle changes have historically been the major factors in the betterment of our health status. And it's likely these non-medical factors will continue to play a pivotal role in our nation's health in the future. Compared to the general public health efforts, many of the new medical/technological modalities tend to be much more expensive and narrower in their impact.

Prevention in the setting of overall community health, as opposed to clinical preventive medicine, which has its own more limited scope, is essential for the long-range success of any universal coverage plan. I'm not referring to "Putting Prevention Into Practice," the catchy phrase used to promote clinical preventive medicine. I've been an active proponent of that approach for almost 30 years. What I'm talking about is, rather, "Putting Prevention Into America." This more comprehensive brand of prevention deserves a much greater role in America's more global quest for "good health for all," as opposed to "health care for all."

America has experienced successes in prevention. Smoke-filled rooms are now a rarity in our society. There have been significant strides towards reducing the use of tobacco—despite some recent setbacks in cutting the rate of teen smoking. There

has also been an increased awareness—accompanied by action—
of the effects of environmental factors on our health. Decreases
in deaths from motor vehicle accidents have come from preventive efforts in the form of safer highways and increased seat
belt use. Improved housing as well as safe water and food have
meant better health for Americans. By and large, these advances
have been inspired by public health but have come through the
political arena or as societal changes, and not through medical
science.

However, as a society we have failed so far to come to grips
with how we should deal with a host of chronic diseases—e.g.,
heart disease, strokes, obesity, arthritis, and diabetes. There is
evidence that chronic diseases affect the uninsured much more
adversely than people with coverage. A study by the Center
for Studying Health System Change[2] found that the uninsured
with chronic illnesses are three times more likely not to get the
medical care they need. Meanwhile, there is a growing body of
evidence that chronic diseases are preventable through lifestyle
modifications. A prospective study published in February 2002[3]
demonstrated that a program of moderate exercise and weight
reduction led to a 58 percent decrease in the incidence of type 2
diabetes. Chronic diseases take a huge economic and human toll
on the American people because so many millions of Americans
suffer from them.

American society has evolved in a manner that has encouraged our current "epidemic" of chronic diseases. Part of the fault
in our failure to deal effectively with chronic diseases through
lifestyle changes (exercise, weight loss, quitting smoking, etc.)
probably comes from having too much faith in medical science.
Curative medicine has done wonders and is often capable of
erasing many of our sins—at a price. If popping a pill can
control your diabetes or clean the fat out of your arteries, why
worry about being a couch potato? I had a patient who, after
his quadruple cardiac bypass surgery, continued to smoke four
packs of cigarettes a day and shun exercise. Why worry, when
an artery can be reamed out with microsurgery? But medical
science, which has provided antidotes for our own self-abuse,
is only partially to blame.

As the speaker at the preventive medicine meeting stated, exercise has not yet become "mainstream" in America. In contrast, limiting the use of tobacco products has, as has the exposure to other environmental toxins. An article on transportation goals in Idaho's Treasure Valley (the area around Boise) appeared in *The Idaho Statesman* in December 2001. The "ambitious goal" in a 20-year plan for commuting was to get people out of their cars. For the "bike or walk" objective, the planners projected *no* growth. Three percent today. And for 20 years hence, still three percent. Reality? Maybe, but it's illustrative of the problem. As a society, we're clueless.

A Prime Example: America's Epidemic of Obesity

Anna is an 11-year-old Hispanic girl brought into the office by her mother with cramping abdominal pains and constipation. She is 4'8" and weighs 140 pounds. Her only physical activity occurs twice a week in her fifth grade physical education class. When at home, she watches "lots" of TV. Her diet includes "a lot" of candy and soda pop. A schoolmate, Marjorie, is nine years old, in fourth grade, and weighs 177 pounds. Her only exercise is two sessions of P.E. a week; she consumes "munchies" and watches TV when she's at home. Her mother developed diabetes at a young age (35) and worries that Marjorie will too.

Our growing epidemic of obesity is a prime example of our society's failure to address the changing American diet and to make exercise "mainstream." Between 1991 and 2000, the prevalence of obesity in American adults increased by 61 percent—to 19.8 percent of all adults. The prevalence of morbid obesity—a body-mass index (BMI) of 40 or more—more than doubled in the same nine years, from 0.9 percent to 2.1 percent.[4]

Internationally, we are winning first place in the contest for the fattest nation. For the 24 OECD developed nations, the U.S. ranks number one—by far—in obesity for both men and women.[5]

Our society is paying a price for the huge increase in obesity, which also leads to more diabetes, heart disease, and worn-out joints. Now we're even seeing kids with type 2 diabetes, something we never saw 20 years ago. In December 2001, The U.S. Surgeon General came out with a report that attributed 300,000 deaths a year to obesity. He blamed most of the disaster on our increasingly sedentary lifestyle. Maybe people figure it doesn't really matter because they can always get insulin pumps, heart bypass grafts, organ transplants, or joint replacements. In the future, maybe people will be able to have beta-cell transplants (for diabetes), gene therapy, and mechanical hearts. But that line of thinking makes no logical (or economic) sense. Maybe, however, it helps to make us complacent. Something has happened to America to make us a sedentary nation. Why have we become so exercise-averse?

Paradoxically, we have seen an increase in the number of recreational centers in America—places where middle-class folks go to "work out." We seem to have spawned a subclass of exercise freaks who do workouts in gyms and run marathons. But the great bulk of Americans, notably those who have lower incomes or must work at more than one job to make ends meet, don't partake in the gym rituals. It's all part of the growing disparities in America, disparities based on economics that translate into heath status disparities.

There are many factors in American life, factors that have influenced our diet and our level of physical activity, that have accelerated our slide, as a nation, to "Fat City." Among them:

1) Literally, Fat City. The urbanization and/or suburbanization of American society.

2) Television and video games. Watching the football games instead of playing touch football, etc. With the exception of a growing elite (e.g., the marathoners and triatheletes), Americans are primarily into spectator sports. And while we watch, we eat.

3) Our dependence on the automobile—and our almost rabid protection of it as a way of life. I recall a letter to

the editor while I was running for public office. Since it was widely known that I rode a bicycle, the writer attacked me, saying the "only way they'd get [him] to stop driving is when they peeled his dead hands off the steering wheel." With this kind of attitude as almost an axiom of American culture, we've seen barely more than token efforts to expand transportation systems based on human power. And we've built our communities in such a spread-out fashion as to make automobile use almost mandatory.

4) Lower wages for working-class people. There are fewer high-paying manufacturing jobs. More people are now working at lower-paying service jobs. Thus, they need to work longer and/or do several jobs. The result: no time or energy left to exercise. There's no time to walk somewhere. And time pressures necessitate using a car.

5) The decrease of physical education in the schools. Too many other demands. Meanwhile, kids in schools have easy access to candy and pop machines.[6]

6) The dominance of team sports (can lead to more joint replacements later) instead of lifetime sports.

7) Despite the increasing availability of "low-fat" foods, Americans, and especially low-income Americans, are taking in more calories. Low incomes and less time combine to increase the consumption of "fast foods." Compared to other countries, food—especially high-carbohydrate food—is cheap in America. One only needs to go to a buffet restaurant and observe plates piled six inches high with food to appreciate the American appetite. Even in non-buffet restaurants, the portion sizes have become humongous. We now have 44 ounce "Big Gulps" and "Colossal Burgers."

8) The commercialization of food, especially on TV. People are bombarded with TV ads selling a plethora of high-calorie snacks, drinks, etc. Food has become part of our American psyche—just as exercise has not.[7]

What Are the Side Effects
of Making Exercise "Mainstream"?

IN ALL FAIRNESS TO America and Americans' attitude towards exercise, there has been some progress in how we look at exercise. The week after the people at the New Orleans hotel confiscated my bike (I got it back, of course), I rode it to another conference at a Marriott hotel in Portland, Oregon. I had biked 11 miles in a pouring rain, and my Gore-tex suit was soaked. The hotel folks at the entryway invited me to put my bike and rain clothes in the valet's room next to the entrance to dry out. What a difference.

I suspect the exercise "gap" in America is part of the larger picture of health disparities, predominantly based on economic class and economic realities. But if we each took some positive action towards creating a society that really valued exercise, we could make real changes, much as we have with smoking and the environment. These changes do not have to take generations to work. They can be accomplished in decades if we have the will. For example, two simple strategies to lessen our dependence upon our automobiles would be: (a) increased investment in mass transit, and (b) making human-powered transportation safe, as with bike trails that connect so that commuting to work can be practical.

Unfortunately, the health care industry's "mainstream" players, with a few notable exceptions, are unlikely to profit from a paradigm shift in how America looks at exercise—or how we improve our diets. The pharmaceutical industry would be especially affected. With the growing epidemic of obesity, the drug companies can look forward to a financial windfall. Many millions of Americans will be taking their "statin" drugs to lower their cholesterol levels. And they could each be spending $3 a day, or $1100 a year, for the rest of their lives. There are the similarly expensive "lifetime" drugs for diabetes, hypertension, and heart disease. People will be buying a wide variety of new look-alike but possibly safer (and more expensive) medications for pains in their stressed-out joints. The profit potential for safe new weight-reduction drugs is also phenomenal. And then there is the panoply of extraordinarily expensive medications, sometimes at

several thousand dollars a dose, that accompany high-tech surgeries like the placement of cardiac stents or transplants. If I were
a drug company CEO looking out for the financial welfare of my
stockholders, I'd worry about exercise becoming "mainstream"
in America. Ironically, his stockholders are probably the same
people who can be found working out at the gyms.

I recently made an exercise-based suggestion to a sales "rep"
from one of the large pharmaceutical corporations. He was at a
diabetes meeting where he was marketing his company's drugs
for diabetes and cholesterol. The latter has annual sales in the
billions. I suggested that his company had a way to demonstrate
just how much they really cared about the health of Americans. I
proposed that his company donate a few billion dollars towards
the promotion of community-oriented exercise in this country.
Media campaigns. Funds for P.E. in schools. Support for modifications in our transportation infrastructure to make human-powered commuting safe and practical. He thought it was a great
idea. We actually will be working on it, but I won't be holding my
breath until it happens.

Exercise as a national norm would likely also negatively
affect the incomes of certain medical specialists, like cardiolo-
gists, cardiac surgeons, and endocrinologists. Orthopedists could
probably break even, as sports injuries could take the place of
what they earn replacing worn-out joints. At least their job would
be more varied. Access to care would be easier, since doctors'
offices wouldn't be so crowded with people who have diabetes,
hypertension, obesity, and depression—the diagnoses that make
up most of the practice of adult medicine. And hospitals and
nursing homes would likely see census decreases as a result of a
generally healthier population. Since exercise has a beneficial
effect on mental health, especially depression, there would be
less need to take care of depression medically, and there would be
less demand on our inadequate mental health system. However,
the drug companies would suffer. A year's treatment for depression with one drug typically costs about $1000.

As for the insurance industry and the HMOs (assuming a
status quo), they could come out ahead. They would pay out less

money for procedures and medications because people would generally be healthier. With fewer "high-risk" people to avoid, they would be able to enroll more people in their plans. Prevention has traditionally received great "lip service" from the HMOs, but more often than not has been used primarily as a marketing tool. They have used the clinical preventive medicine measures (e.g., immunization rates) largely to sell their products. There has been little commitment (with some exceptions, as with Group Health of Puget Sound and their promotion of bicycle helmets) to change the way society looks at prevention in general.

Action Steps to "Put Prevention Into America"

WHAT HAS BEEN LACKING overall is real advocacy, in the form of personal commitment and financial support, for real prevention (exercise and diet modification being prime examples). Compared to the amount of money, the many billions of dollars, that go into the marketing of poor health habits by the "dark side" of American business, prevention gets a pittance. Even physicians, hassled by paperwork and tied up in their hectic daily routines, don't have the time or the foresight to "get involved" in actions that would really help their communities—and thereby their patients. But industry can find millions to sell Pepsi in schools or promote the "statin" drugs that lower cholesterol.

Real prevention could go a long way to making America a much more humane society. What if we had a society with a higher degree of wellness? That could, of course, go along with a narrowing of the disparities between the well and the unwell in America, disparities that generally correlate with economic class. What if we had less stress in our society? Would our health indicators improve? What if we put more value on well-being than fancy homes, cars, and maximizing profits? Compare a one-and-a-half hour drive to work in stop-and-go traffic on an L.A. freeway with a ten-minute bike ride to work in a small town in the Midwest. Time spent talking on the phone in an office cubicle versus time spent doing physical work in the outdoors. Or having a modest dwelling and time to spend with family, as opposed to not having the family time—or the time to exercise—because long hours of work are required to meet high mortgage payments.

There are, of course, the direct positive health effects of exercise, and how these affect our overall humanity. We relate better to each other if we're not depressed, not sick, not limping with a worn-out knee joint, and more able to do our daily activities for others and ourselves. Our physical and mental well-being is directly related to physical activity. Yet exercise is still a "fringe" activity for the majority of Americans. What can we do, as individuals and as a society, to make prevention "real" in America? To cause a paradigm shift in how America looks at prevention, and (more specifically) exercise?[8] Some practical action steps include:

1) Convince American industry to invest in the promotion of prevention, especially to try to integrate exercise into the daily lives of Americans, including at the workplace. A practical example is the convenient placement of stairs—versus elevators.

2) Governmental support for the same (1), funded at no extra cost through cost-shifting away from sedentary transportation to human-powered transportation.

3) Urban planning that makes human-powered transportation practical and safe.

4) Increased physical education in schools, with an emphasis on lifetime physical activities, combined with a movement to have only healthy foods in schools.

5) Increased community-based efforts, with financial support from the private and public sectors, to promote physical activity for families, communities, and individuals.

6) Encouragement and participation of community leaders, including politicians and health professionals, in exercise-based activities that are not primarily competitive.

7) Increased public health outreach activities, especially in schools and in communities, to promote healthy lifestyles, especially physical activity and a healthy diet.

8) Appropriate taxation (or the opposite, positive financial incentives) to encourage healthy lifestyles, especially exercise as a routine activity. Examples: greatly increased tobacco, alcohol and gasoline taxes; taxing soft drinks; higher vehicle licensing fees. Conversely, subsidies and/or rewards for people who walk or bike to work, agricultural subsidies for the producers of fruits and vegetables—as opposed to the current subsidies for producers of tobacco and sugar.

9) A national campaign, looked at as "an investment in America," to promote prevention and exercise as goals that will improve our society's health and sense of well-being as well as make health care for everybody more affordable.

10) Research activities to document the effects of "Putting Prevention into America" and making it truly mainstream.

As a matter of public policy, it makes unequivocal economic sense, for all the many reasons outlined above, to support efforts at all levels to make exercise "mainstream" in America. "Putting Prevention into America," with the objective of making prevention, and especially physical activity, a new paradigm, will serve our nation well. Replacing the current paradigm that places a blind faith in medical science to "fix everything" would be a huge step forward. It would also be a key measure going "beyond universal coverage" to improve the health of Americans. It would make us a healthier and kinder society. And it would help make "Health Care for All" an affordable reality, not just a dream.

Summary of Key Points

- We have an epidemic of obesity in America, largely due to an increasingly sedentary lifestyle and poor eating habits.

- We are the "fattest" nation of all the developed countries.

- Unless we deal effectively with obesity and our lack of physical activity, we will see an ever-larger increase in chronic diseases such as diabetes, high blood pressure, heart problems, and strokes.

- We must strive to make physical activity "mainstream" in America.

- The long-term financial consequences of failing to deal with preventive measures will severely affect our ability to create an affordable health care system.

WILCOX'S **ANTI-CORPULENE PILLS!**

A NEW DISCOVERY IN MEDICINE.

POSITIVELY REDUCES SUPERFLUOUS FLESH 15 POUNDS A MONTH.

Cause No Sickness, Contain No Poisons, and NEVER FAIL.

"I have lost nearly one-half pound a day, or nearly thirty pounds in eight weeks." MRS. JAS. A. McCOLLUM, South Argyle, N. Y.

"I lost five pounds the first five days that I used Anti-Corpulene Pills, and four pounds the next five days." MISS JENNIE DALBY, Dalby Springs, Texas.

"I have lost forty pounds, feel ten years younger, and would not be back where I was last Summer for $1,000." MRS. R. E. DIBBLE, Ju.. Summit, N. Y.

Hundreds of equally wonderful results. Send 4 cts. for Circulars and voluntary testimonials of grateful patients.

WILCOX SPECIFIC CO., PHILADELPHIA, PA.

Chapter 18

Epilogue: Beyond Universal Coverage

Marian is the single mother of a teenager diagnosed with a bipolar disorder. Even though her employer provided health insurance, she was forced to leave a job of 11 years so that her son could receive Medicaid. She worried that her son might require extended hospitalization for his problem. If that happened, under her old insurance, which covered only a maximum of eight days in the hospital, she would have had to pay the balance, probably tens of thousands of dollars out of pocket. At one point, her son's psychiatrist suggested that Marian turn over custody of her son to the state so he could be placed in a shelter home and thereby get Medicaid.

Marian had also been turned over to collection agencies by physicians who wouldn't accept payments. And she had to beg hospitals to write off parts of bills to avoid bankruptcy. When her son recently broke his jaw, her insurance would pay only 50 percent of the bill because the surgeon was not a "preferred provider." The insurance company failed to tell her that no pediatric surgeons in Idaho had agreed to be "preferred providers."

UNIVERSAL COVERAGE ALONE IS not sufficient to reach the "desired outcome" of good health for everyone in America. But we can look at national health insurance or Health Care for All as a type of incremental change. A major step forward, but not a panacea for all that ails our health care system. It would be a boon for access to care. It would be undoubtedly the most essential

234

step in decreasing health care disparities in America. But it wouldn't necessarily guarantee access, let alone good quality care. Look at Medicaid, for example. People with Medicaid—and Medicaid can have a very comprehensive benefit package—often have a difficult time finding physicians. Finding a dentist who will take Medicaid is more difficult yet. For those with Medicare, there is sometimes a problem with access, while minority Americans with Medicare have been shown to get less care.

Besides the lack of insurance coverage and/or financial barriers, there are other factors that affect the ability of Americans to get the health care they need. Those other obstacles include geographical access, cultural and linguistic barriers, shortages or maldistribution of certain kinds of health professionals (e.g., nurses, dentists, and mental health workers), and even racism.[1] In addition, there are questions related to the scientific appropriateness of the care delivered. Transportation can be a major problem, as can a host of social circumstances that have an impact on health.

Community health centers like to think that they are "the specialists" in dealing with these "peripheral" but essential circumstances that affect the ability to get needed care. And, indeed, the health centers do represent more than just a "safety net" for the uninsured because of the "extra" services they provide. Even Canada, with its universal coverage, has community health centers to serve those "special" populations. Beyond coverage, to serve the health care needs of America, our system will need to address such issues as improving our information systems, increasing the practice of evidence-based medicine, eliminating medical errors, and taking more accountability for outcomes. We will also need to give increased attention to prevention—especially in the sweeping sense of societal change—without which we will continue to fall short in our pursuit of good health. We'll need to give a higher priority to such issues as pop machines and physical education in schools, versus designing protocols for the use of cholesterol-lowering drugs. Deciding which people need their carotid arteries reamed out is important, but it makes much more sense to invest more of our resources in finding ways to provide kids with positive alternatives to watching TV and playing video games.

Assuring Adequate Coverage

UNIVERSAL COVERAGE MUST INCLUDE a comprehensive and adequate package of benefits that meets the health care needs of all Americans or it will be a "sham" endeavor. At the very least, it must cover inpatient and outpatient care, emergency care, mental health, diagnostic and lab tests, long-term care, basic dental and eye care, pharmaceuticals, adequate home health services, and necessary medical equipment.

At our evening clinic, I saw a middle-aged Mexican-American man who had brought in his daughter for an earache. As I finished giving him instructions on what to do for his daughter, he pulled out a sheaf of papers and asked if I could give an opinion. What he showed me was a health insurance policy for which he was paying $39 a month. Its main benefit was $50 a day for hospitalizations. Was this man insured? I wonder if he was one of the people polled by the Census Bureau when they calculated the number of uninsured Americans.

Then there is the issue of deductibles and co-pays, which has been addressed earlier (see Chapter 6)—the "personal responsibility" smokescreen. Of course, we should all exercise more, drink less, wear our seat belts and not smoke at all. But all those obvious measures are not why the experts and the corporate types are pushing "personal responsibility." They're promoting it because they want a sweet-sounding excuse for shifting costs to the patient/employee. For less well-to-do patients, shifted costs often mean delaying or omitting care—even when it's necessary. It means a multi-tiered system, where the rich get one kind of care, the poor get another. Guess who would get the plan that has more comprehensive and timely care with fewer barriers?

There is an inconsistency in the call for outcome accountability and the use of scientific methods with the promotion of "personal responsibility" in the form of higher costs for patients. As mentioned above, I don't know of any scientific evidence showing that deductibles and co-pays produce better outcomes.

Nor am I aware of studies proving that even higher deductibles and co-pays bring even better results.

Perhaps the health policy wonks, in their wisdom, have concluded that the use or overuse of services (whether necessary or not) is a risky affair. They may, not without some reason, fear that the very use of services will generate a certain degree of iatrogenic (self-caused) bad outcomes. But I don't think they have that much insight, and I do think it's all about money and short-term savings that accrue to employers and insurers, as opposed to patients or employees. Again, there is a lack of appreciation for the fact that delayed or omitted care costs more for everybody in the long run. The bottom line: any universal coverage plan must deal with the problem of deductibles and co-pays so that access to care for people with marginal incomes, as well as middle-class people, is not adversely affected.

Reclaiming Dignity

THE NEW SYSTEM MUST allow people dignity. How people are treated and how they feel about themselves is important. A system of universal coverage with everyone in the same risk pool would eliminate the stigma that goes with Medicaid and the degree of disdain or rejection that some people with Medicaid (and the uninsured) must currently endure. Real universal coverage, as opposed to a stratified multi-tiered system that allowed the rich one kind of care and the poor another, would help return a sense of dignity to individuals. It's the same kind of dignity that Medicare provides for our elderly population. Only it would be better, since Medicare has evolved into an incomplete system. Universal coverage would help restore a sense of dignity to our nation. In the eyes of the rest of the world, America has become ethically "tainted" because of our failure to provide health insurance for everyone, as they do in all the other developed countries.

I was sitting next to a Canadian on a flight to Seattle a few years ago. We talked a bit about health care, and he said, "You know, I admire you Americans for many things, but, for the life of me, I can't understand why you don't have universal cover-

age." I've talked to Europeans who think we're barbaric because
we actually allow someone to go bankrupt because he or she had
the misfortune to be sick or injured. It amazes me that we've
become so clueless to the fundamental issues surrounding health
care that well-meaning Americans, who consider themselves
as caring beings, can sense nothing wrong about saying, "I think
it's okay that Americans who can afford health care can get it,
whereas those who aren't able to afford it can't."

Keeping America Clueless

THE MEDICAL-INDUSTRIAL COMPLEX HAS a financial stake
in keeping America clueless about how our health system fails us
as individuals and as a nation. We spend more—40 percent more
than the next most expensive country—on health care, yet reap
mediocre results as a population, results that rank us in the mid-
twenties for most health indicators (see page 149). We get poor
value for all our spending. Yet we Americans have been conned
into believing that "we have the best health system in the world,"
along with a host of other myths (see Chapter 1). The mythology
is not accidental. The spreading and maintenance of the myths
has been bankrolled by the vested interests. The millions spent by
the AMA in the early '90s to discredit Canada's system, the many
more millions spent in 2000 by the pharmaceutical industry
on "the bus from Canada," and the millions spent on "Harry
and Louise" by the insurance industry and small business to
kill Clinton's plan (bad as it was) are but a few examples of the
concerted and directed effort to kill or delay meaningful health
care reform.

These efforts to keep America clueless have been amazingly
successful—to the point of having created inner (almost) dogmas
that inhibit rational thought. This programmed mythology has
implanted certain catchwords in our collective American psyche.
In seemingly rational discussions about health care, throwing in
a phrase like "socialized medicine," "the federal government,"
"rationing," "taxes," "Great Britain," or "Canada" brings discussion to a screeching halt. Minds close. Even "universal coverage"

and "health care reform" have become equated with socialism, and Americans certainly don't want *that*.

The issue of health care in America has become so complex that a few million media dollars to plant doubt can block significant change. Part of the ease in derailing new ideas comes from the relative lack of involvement of Americans in health care as an issue. Unless someone is ill or injured, there is little interaction with the system or appreciation for how it *doesn't* work.

The degree of cluelessness is amazing. It envelops our citizenry, much of the media, health care professionals, politicians, and the health care industry in general. It even touches many of the health policy gurus, who, in their academic world of ecnomic theory, often have little sense of what it means to lose your dignity in a dysfunctional health care system. Only after they've been sick and had the misfortune to experience the crazy side of American health care, as did Paul Ellwood (one of the original chief gurus of managed care), do they wake up and realize something has gone wrong. Many thinking people, including consultants and people from the insurance industry who have worked in health care for decades, appreciate the need for meaningful reform with "one risk pool." Most of them are of the mind that we need to go through more pain (i.e., more futile incremental or piecemeal approaches) before there will be a more general recognition of the need for truly universal coverage with one risk pool.

Although the events of 9/11 reminded us of our potential to share some values as a community, it will take a stronger sense of "community responsibility" (as opposed to "personal responsibility") to assure every person in America access to health care. Even in the face of strong economic arguments for universal coverage—every study done shows it would save us money—there is reluctance to bite the bullet and move forward. Whenever the moneyed interests perceive a threat to their empires, they spring to action to befuddle us and keep us clueless—as they tried to do with the November 2001 Portland, Maine, referendum for single-payer health care reform. The

vested interests lost that referendum, but they'll be back to protect their "bottom lines" and keep us clueless.

The Global Picture

THE AMERICAN QUANDARY WITH Health Care for All, as well as
the looming "meltdown" of our health care system, is really only
a part of the larger picture. At the beginning of the 21st Century,
a worldwide struggle is taking place over the role of "globalization." In polarizing terms, the conflict could be described as one
between the multinational corporations and the working people
of the world. Of course, that's too simple a definition. But it does
come down to a battle between the "haves" and the "have-nots,"
with the "haves" telling the "have-nots" they should have faith in
free markets, capitalism, privatization, free trade, etc. Around the
world, the efforts of the International Monetary Fund—notably
their "structural readjustment" or privatization plans—have
had disastrous results for working people. The rich have gotten
richer, and the poor poorer. A recent example of the effects of
privatization gone awry is the economic collapse in Argentina.
Ironically, Argentina used to have a respected and responsive
publicly administered health care system. Much of that system
has now been privatized, resulting in markedly decreased access
to health care for most Argentines.

What's happening in America's health care system today is,
of course, influenced by the kind of thinking that has occurred
with the world's shift towards globalization. The value conflicts
are similar. The private vs. public arguments. Health care as a
right vs. "the market."

Health care cannot really be viewed in a vacuum. It inter-
relates with other social and economic issues, such as poverty,
hunger, racism, a living wage, adequate housing, and education.
In a larger context, our current dilemma with health care raises
the whole issue of whether, as a community, we have some
responsibility to care for each other—as opposed to "personal
responsibility." This "community responsibility" question applies
to all the other problem social issues as well. On a perhaps more

radical bent, some, including author Barbara Ehrenreich, have asserted, "The 'working poor'...are in fact the major philanthropists of our society. They neglect their own children so the children of others will be cared for...."[2] The inequities and disparities in health care are perhaps the most egregious shortcoming of American society today because of the huge impact they have on so many millions of people.

Unless there is some reversal of direction soon, America's health care seems to be headed increasingly towards greater discrepancies between rich and poor as we progressively become a "culture of extreme inequality."[3] We seem to be lacking leadership as we drift towards a multi-tiered health care system. A system where the very rich will receive "concierge care," while the poor could be relegated to a phone card that will give them an hour a month of consultation with a "Dial-a-Nurse" service in Minneapolis or Bangalore.

Steps We Must Take as a Responsible Nation to Improve the Health of Our Communities

IF WE ARE TO MOVE forward, "right the wrong," make health care affordable and accessible for every person in America, improve the health of our nation, and remedy the loss of dignity that we have inflicted on ourselves as individuals and as a nation, there are some specific actions we need to take.

1) As the first step—and one without which the rest will be more difficult to implement—we must have universal coverage. Everybody in, nobody out.

2) That universal coverage needs to be based on a "single risk pool" or it will *de facto* not be truly universal, as it will be gamed to exclude people who are high risk. Without the "single risk pool" there will be a multitiered system with its inherent inequities.

3) We need a paradigm shift in how we deal with health care and health. A change from the curative to the preventive. We currently overfund the curative and seriously

underfund the preventive—perhaps by a ratio of 100:1. "Preventive" must include not just clinical preventive measures, but also strive for more comprehensive societal change (with the adequate allocation of resources). It's not just "putting prevention into practice." It's putting prevention into life.

4) Part of that prevention is minimizing delayed care and health care disparities. The key measure to reach these goals is universal coverage, but there are other barriers that must be addressed as well (see above).

5) Health care needs to return to an emphasis on health, not cost or profit. It should be regarded as a "public good," not a commodity. The pursuit of profit through health care produces twisted incentives that only lead to poorer outcomes, injustice, and discrimination. The goal should be health, not wealth. In the process, we need to assure that the quality of that health care is good and that our nation receives good value for what we spend on health care.

6) There should be grassroots efforts to (a) define community priorities, (b) assure community involvement and action, and (c) inform the clueless. The American people should understand who the "modern-day snake oil merchants" are and what motivates them.

7) Harry and Louise should be recruited away from the "Dark Side" of health care and be used nationwide to combat the merchants of misinformation and myth.

8) Instead of using the mantra of "personal responsibility" to blame the victims, we should place a much higher value on "community responsibility" and restoring personal dignity. We also need to assure "corporate responsibility" in health care—or have them convert to a not-for-profit status—an idea that needs to be explored seriously.

9) The system needs to be simplified, not made more complex. Complexity is a barrier in itself.

10) As a nation, we need to recognize that national health insurance or Health Care for All is good for the American economy, perhaps the only way to avoid the meltdown of our health care system, and (most important) the "right thing to do." Health Care for All will help not only individuals, but also our nation, regain the dignity we have lost because of our health care system's egregious inequities and shortcomings.

Summary of Key Points

- Universal coverage (or Health Care for All) is only the first step towards a larger goal: good health for all.

- The benefit package must be comprehensive and adequate enough to address the real health care needs of all Americans.

- We must educate all Americans about health and health care to counter the efforts of the medical-industrial complex to "keep America clueless."

- We need to give more importance to "community responsibility" as opposed to "personal responsibility."

- Health care should be regarded as a "public good," not a commodity.

- There are many other factors that we will need to address in order to assure good health for everyone—including poverty, racism, education, decent housing, a living wage, the scientific basis of medicine, and effective prevention.

- Without Health Care for All, we will not regain our dignity as a nation.

I'M FROM THE

Anidrosis

Sanitarium !

TO

Alleviate Suffering Humanity by Smoth-
ering the Germs of DISEASE in
COMPOUND VAPOR FUMIGATION.

All Obstructive Elements secreted to
the defeat of nature promptly eliminated
and disinfection assured, thus allowing
Mother Nature to put on her reconstruc-
tive work.

GREAT BOON FOR RHEUMATICS

Afterword

IT SEEMS ENIGMATIC that we have by far the greatest resources for health care of all nations on earth, yet we fall far short of other industrialized nations on measures of universality, coverage and access. And we have one of the least equitable systems, both in the way we fund health care and in the way that we allocate our health care resources.

In *Health Care Meltdown* Bob LeBow explains how we arrived at this state. But even more importantly, he explains precisely what we can do about it. He shows us how we can provide truly comprehensive care for everyone with no significant increase in health care spending.

So how close are we to realizing Bob's model of an ideal system of funding health care? Since he finished writing this book, the numbers of uninsured have continued to increase. Costs are continuing to escalate well in excess of inflation, thereby threatening affordability even for those who are insured.

And what has been our response? Employers are shifting more of the premium costs to their employees. Insurers are decreasing the benefits covered by their plans and are increasing the out-of-pocket cost sharing for their beneficiaries. States are slashing their budgets and with them the health care programs for those who cannot afford to purchase their own insurance or pay for their care. The federal government has responded by introducing health savings accounts that provide tax advantages for higher-income individuals, but concentrate lower-income individuals with greater health care needs into traditional plans. This drives the premium up to unaffordable levels, and leaves those with the greatest needs with intolerable financial exposure.

Relatively healthy individuals still fare well under the current system since they face primarily higher premiums but are spared of the other costs. But those with severe acute or chronic disorders are finding their coverage to be inadequate and the out-of-pocket costs unaffordable. Our non-system of private plans, public programs, and no-programs-at-all is failing us miserably.

Bob's message to us is more crucial than ever. We can provide affordable, comprehensive health care for everyone. We need only to look at the deteriorating coverage of today and ask ourselves: What would Bob say? Fortunately, in *Health Care Meltdown* he has provided us with the answer. Now we must act on it.

Don McCanne, M.D.
2002 & 2003 president of
Physicians for a National Health Program
www.pnhp.org
February 2004

Notes

Selected Bibliography

Appendix

Glossary of Terms

Index

Dr. E. Smith's,
PATENT
MAGNETIC
INDUCTOR.

If not called for in 10 days P. M. return to
Dr. E. SMITH, Normal, Ills.

Notes

INTRODUCTION

1. See: <www.coveringtheuninsured.org>

2. Health economist Uwe Reinhardt used this term when he described what some parents were forced to become in order to get care for their children in: Reinhardt, Uwe E., PhD. "Wanted: A Clearly Articulated Social Ethic for American Health Care." *JAMA* 278(17) (November 5, 1997): 1446-1447.

3. Bob Kerry. Testimony before the Senate Finance Committee on "The Administration's FY 2003 Budget Proposals for Prescription Drugs." (March 7, 2002).

CHAPTER 1

1. Bezruchka, Stephen, MD. "Is Our Society Making You Sick?" *Newsweek,* (February 26, 2001): p.14.

2. Starfield, Barbara, MD, MPH. "Is U.S. Health Care Really the Best in the World?" *JAMA* 284(4). (October 25, 2000): 483-485.

3. World Health Organization. *The World Health Report 2000. Health Systems: Improving Performance.* Geneva. (2000).

4. "Emergency Care 'Safety Net' Unraveling." *U.S.A. Today,* (February 4-6, 2000).

5. Available at <www.acponline.org/uninsured/>.

6. Kaiser Family Foundation. "Sicker and Poorer: The Consequences of Being Uninsured." (May 2002). <www.kff.org>.

7. Institute of Medicine. *Care Without Coverage: Too Little, Too Late.* National Academy Press. (2002).

8. Corlin, Richard F., MD. "The time is right to fix the problem of the uninsured." *American Medical News,* (January 21, 2002).

249

9. See: Grumbach, Kevin, MD. "Insuring the Uninsured. Time to End the Aura of Invisibility." *JAMA* 284(16) (October 25, 2000): 2114-2116.

10. Quinn, Jane Bryant. "The Invisible Uninsured." *Newsweek,* (March 1, 1999).

11. Garrett, Laurie. *Betrayal of Trust: The Collapse of Global Public Health.* Hyperion. New York. (2000).

12. Kleinke, J.D. *Oxymorons: The Myth of the U.S. Health Care System.* Jossey-Bass. (2001).

13. Personal communication, (December 13, 2001).

14. Our Community Health Center serves a total of about 18,000 patients in southwest Idaho. Our staff includes eight physicians and eight mid-levels (nurse practitioners and physician assistants). We have a large number of patients with diabetes because our population is about half Hispanic.

15. Organization for Economic Cooperation and Development. *OECD Health Data 2000.* Paris. OECD. (2000). The U.S. estimate for 2002 is 14.7 percent of our GDP.

16. Ibid.

17. Light, Donald. "Health Care for All: A Conservative Case." *Commonweal,* (February 22, 2002).

18. Armstrong, Pat; Armstrong, Hugh; with Fegan, Claudia, MD. *Universal Health Care. What the United States Can Learn from the Canadian Experience.* The New Press, New York. (1998).

19. Personal communication from health economist Donald W. Light through "Quote of the Day." (March 2002). Available through <www.pnhp.org>.

20. Ibid. (May 5, 2002).

21. Wielawski, Irene. "Gouging the Medically Uninsured: A Tale of Two Bills." *Health Affairs* 19(5). (September/October 2000): 180-185.

22. See: <www.kff.org>.

23. "Prescription Drug Trends." Henry J. Kaiser Family Foundation. Washington, DC. (July 2000).

24. "Prescription Drugs Policy Toolkit." Center for Policy Alternatives.

25. U.S. Department of Health and Human Services. "Securing the Benefits of Medical Innovation for Seniors: The Role of Prescription Drugs and Drug

Coverage." <aspe.hhs.gov/health/reports/medicalinnovation/> (July 2002). The report defends the pricing and profits of U.S. drug manufacturers.

26. Little, Shannon. "Public Citizen Report Debunks R&D Myths." *Public Citizen News*, (September/October 2001).

27. This phenomenon is described in an article: Gerth, Jeff and Stolberg, Sheryl Gay. "Drug Companies Profit From Research Supported by Taxpayers." *The New York Times,* (April 23, 2000).

28. The Associated Press. "States: Drug Maker Delayed Generics." *The Idaho Statesman,* (June 5, 2002). Taxol was discovered by the National Cancer Institute, which licensed the drug to Bristol-Myers.

29. Stolberg, Sheryl Gay and Gerth, Jeff. "How Companies Stall Generics and Keep Themselves Healthy." *The New York Times*, (July 23, 2000).

30. A similar situation exists for the middlemen who do group purchasing of medical supplies for hospitals. See Chapter 2, "Ignorance of the Costs."

31. For accounts of these practices, see: <www.nofreelunch.org> and Mueller, Rudolph, MD. *As Sick As It Gets.* Chapter 4. "The Pharmaceutical Companies." Olin Frederick, Inc., Dunkirk, NY. (2001).

32. Angell, Marcia, MD. "The Pharmaceutical Industry – To Whom Is It Accountable?" *New England Journal of Medicine* 342(25) (June 22, 2000): 1902-1904.

33. Davis, Karen, "Universal Coverage in the United States: Lessons from Experience of the 20th Century," *Journal of Urban Health: Bulletin of the New York Academy of Medicine* 78 (March 2001): 46-58.

34. Mofidi, Mahyar, DMD, MPH; Rozier, R. Gary, DDS, MPH; King, Rebecca S., DDS, MPH. "Problems With Access to Care for Medicaid-Insured Children: What Caregivers Think." *American Journal of Public Health* 92(1) (January 2002): 53.

35. Rosenbaum, Sara, JD. "Medicaid." *New England Journal of Medicine* 346 (February 21, 2002): 635-640.

36. Pear, Robert. "9 of 10 Nursing Homes in U.S. Lack Adequate Staff, a Government Study Finds." *The New York Times,* (February 18, 2002).

37. Reinhardt, Uwe, PhD. Speech before National Chamber of Commerce. (October 1999).

38. Broder, David. "Fix Health Care Now." Op-Ed. *The Washington Post,* (January 6, 2002).

39. Ivins, Molly. Creators Syndicate, Inc. column. (March 26, 2002). Ivins adds, "But if you want to see horror in action, try the emergency room of any large public hospital in this country."

CHAPTER 2

1. Elaborating on her "passion" for solving the problem of the uninsured, Ms. Cohen was talking on a panel that took place on April 30, 2002, to discuss House Concurrent Resolution 99, the "Health Care Access Resolution." Ms. Cohen was one of the chief architects of New York's Family Health Plus Program.

2. *Register* Editorial Board. "Editorial: The health-care hodgepodge. A single-payer national plan makes more and more sense." *The Des Moines Register*, (January 4, 2002).

3. Mueller, Rudolph, MD. *As Sick As It Gets*. Olin Frederick, Inc., Dunkirk, NY. (2001).

4. O'Connor, Kathleen, MA. *The Buck Stops Nowhere. Why America's Healthcare is All Dollars and No Sense.* Hara Publishing Company, Seattle. (2001).

5. Feachem, Richard GA, et al. "Getting more for their dollar: A comparison of the NHS with California's Kaiser Permanente." *British Medical Journal* 324 (January 25, 2002): 135-143.

6. However, as Grumbach points out, the British health care system spends less than one-third per capita than the U.S. system, and "...for macro-level economic efficiency, the NHS remains the standard bearer."

7. Reinhardt, Uwe, PhD. "Harness Information to Make Health Care Work." *Managed Care*, (January 2002). He says, "From the perspective of those who pay for health care and of those who use it, our system remains one of the most opaque sectors in the economy."

8. Lankarge, Vicki, for insure.com. Posted on *MSN Money* (February 6, 2002).

9. Bogdanich, Walt. "2 Powerful Groups Hold Sway Over Buying at Many Hospitals." *The New York Times*, (March 4, 2002).

10. Glied, Sherry A. "Challenges and Options for Increasing the Number of Americans with Health Insurance," The Commonwealth Fund. (January 2001): p. 13.

11. Light, Donald. "Health Care for All: A Conservative Case." *Commonweal*, (February 22, 2002).

12. Sparrow, Malcolm K. *License to Steal. How Fraud Bleeds America's Health Care System.* Westview Press. (2000).

13. Asch, SM, Sloss, EM, Hogan, G, Brook, RH, Kravitz, RL. "Measuring underuse of necessary care among elderly Medicare beneficiaries using inpatient and outpatient claims." *JAMA* 284 (2000): 2325-33.

14. Figures from OECD data from 1996. Anderson, Gerard; Hussey, Peter Sotir. "Comparing Health System Performance In OECD Countries." *Health Affairs*, (May/June 2001).

CHAPTER 3

1. Ironically, another new expensive rheumatoid arthritis drug, which was pulled off the market, is now appearing nationally in ads paid for by lawyers preparing a class action suit against the manufacturer for its harmful side effects.

2. See: Katz, Steven J., et al. "Phantoms in the Snow: Canadians' Use of Health Care Services in the United States." *Health Affairs* 21 (3) (May/June 2002): 19-31. In this 1996 study only 20 of 18,000 respondents said they had purposefully gone to the U.S. to obtain any kind of health care.

3. Brown, Gordon. Chancellor of the Exchequer. *The Economist*, (April 13-18, 2002): p. 18.

4. Speaking as a panelist on a discussion of House Concurrent Resolution 99, the "Health Care Access Resolution," (April 30, 2002).

5. Appleby, Julie. "Hospitals fight for turf in medical arms race." *USA Today*, (February 20, 2002).

6. Mandel, Michael J. "Economic Trends: Health Care's Economic Payoff." *Business Week*, (April 29, 2002).

7. Freedman, Michael. "The Tort Mess." *Forbes*, (May 13, 2002): 91-98.

8. Anthony, Joseph. "The Answer for Small Business: Guaranteed Health Care." (December 2001). <www.bcentral.com/articles/anthony/166.asp>

9. Kuttner, Robert. "A Dirty Little Secret: Managed Care is Bad for Business." *Business Week*, (December 21, 1998): p. 18.

10. Wallace, Mike. "Mind and Body." Op-Ed. *The New York Times*, (December 11, 2001).

11. Ellwood, Paul M., Jr., MD. "Does Managed Care Need to Be Replaced?" *Medscape General Medicine*, (October 22, 2001).

12. Ibid.

13. Gail Shearer, Director of Health Policy Analysis for Consumers Union, at a panel discussion on House Concurrent Resolution 99. (April 30, 2002).

14. In 2000.

15. COBRA guarantees some employees continuation of their insurance coverage for 18 months after leaving their jobs, but the employee must pay for the coverage.

CHAPTER 4

1. Altman, Drew. "The Uninsured Find Fewer Doctors in the House." *The New York Times,* (August 30, 1998).

2. See: American College of Physicians-American Society of Internal Medicine. "No Health Insurance? It's Enough to Make You Sick – Scientific Research Linking the Lack of Health Coverage to Poor Health." (2000). <www.acponline.org/uninsured/lack-contents.htm> and Kaiser Family Foundation. "Sicker and Poorer. The Consequences of Being Uninsured." (May 2002). <www.kff.org>

3. Gregg, Edward W., et al. "Use of Diabetes Preventive Care and Complications Risk in Two African-American Communities." *American Journal of Preventive Medicine* 21(3) (October 2001): 197-202.

4. Herbert, Bob. "Hunger in the City." Op-Ed. *The New York Times*, (November 22, 2001).

CHAPTER 5

1. "Second Class Medicine." *Consumer Reports*, (September 2000): 42-50.

2. Ferrer, Robert L., MD, MPH. "A Piece of My Mind. Within the System of No-System." *JAMA* 286(20) (November 28, 2001): 2513-2514.

3. In 2002, 200 percent of poverty is $36,200 for a family of four.

4. Holahan, John; Spillman, Brenda. "Health Care Access for Uninsured Adults: A Strong Safety Net Is Not the Same as Insurance." The Urban Institute. Series B, No. B-42 (January 2002).

CHAPTER 6

1. Rasell, M. Edith, MD. "Cost Sharing in Health Insurance — a Reexamination." *New England Journal of Medicine* 332(17) (April 27, 1995).

2. Evans, R.G.; Barer, M.L; Hertzman, C. "The 20-year Experiment: Accounting For, Explaining, and Evaluating Health Care Cost Containment in Canada and the United States." *Annual Review of Public Health* 12 (1991): 481-518.

3. Tamblyn R, Laprise R, Hanley JA, et al. "Adverse Events Associated with Prescription Drug-Cost Sharing Among Poor and Elderly Persons." *JAMA.* 285 (2001): 421-429.

4. i.e., insurance that paid everything with zero co-pays and deductibles.

CHAPTER 7

1. Sider, Ronald J. *Just Generosity. A New Vision for Overcoming Poverty in America.* Chapter 6: "Does Justice Include Health Care for the Poor?" Baker Books, Grand Rapids, Michigan. (1999).

2. Spoken at a panel discussion of House Concurrent Resolution 99, the "Health Care Access Resolution." (April 30, 2002).

3. See: <www.coveringtheuninsured.org>.

4. Also at the panel discussion of House Concurrent Resolution 99. (April 30, 2002).

5. Friends have told me that, outside conservative rural America, the "WWJD" bumper sticker is unrecognized. But it represents how some religious values have become codified in mainstream America. With respect to health care, I'd like to see it translated as, "What Would Justice Decree?"

CHAPTER 8

1. For a complete discussion of the issue, see: Garrett, Laurie. *Betrayal of Trust: The Collapse of Global Public Health.* Hyperion, New York. (2000).

CHAPTER 9

1. Dao, James. "On the Streets of Baltimore, the Word on Medicare is 'Expand', Not 'Reform'." *The New York Times*, (September 8, 2000).

2. Economic Policy Institute. *Paycheck Economics.* "Medicare at the Crossroads. Vouchers Take Us in the Wrong Direction." (March 2001).

3. Krugman, Paul. "Bad Medicine." Op-Ed. *The New York Times*, (March 19, 2002).

CHAPTER 10

1. David B. Williams, professor of sociology at the University of Michigan, as quoted in *The New York Times*, (March 21, 2002). He was reporting on an Institute of Medicine study showing that minorities, even if they're insured, get inferior care in America. He added, "...This report demonstrates that the playing field [in American health care] clearly is not level."

2. Jacob, Julie A. "Managed Care Looks Abroad." *American Medical News*, (September 6, 1999).

3. All 1998 figures. *OECD Health Data 2000.* OECD. Paris. (2000). For 2000, the U.S. per capita spending on health care was $4637.

4. Light, Donald. "Health Care for All. A Conservative Case." *Commonweal*, (February 22, 2002).

5. Barker, William H., *Adding Life to Years. Organized Geriatrics Services in Great Britain and Implications for the United States.* The Johns Hopkins University Press, Baltimore and London. (1987).

6. Epstein, Randi Hutter, "So Lucky to Give Birth in England." *The New York Times,* Health & Fitness. (December 4, 2001).

7. The myth of the "droves" of Canadians coming south for health care is soundly debunked in a study: Katz, Steven J., et al. "Phantoms in the Snow: Canadians' Use of Health Care in the United States." *Health Affairs* 21(3) (May/June 2002): 19-31. In this study, only 20 of 18,000 respondents said they had gone to the U.S. for the purpose of obtaining any type of health care.

8. Armstrong, Pat; Armstrong, Hugh; with Fegan, Claudia, MD. *Universal Health Care. What the United States Can Learn from the Canadian Experience.* The New Press, New York. (1998).

CHAPTER 11

1. "The Unraveling of Health Insurance." *Consumer Reports*, (July 2002): 48-53.

2. In the past, as in the '90s, estimates of future health care costs have been fraught with error.

3. See: Mandel, Michael J. "Economic Trends: Health Care's Economic Payoff." *Business Week,* (April 29, 2002).

4. See: <www.ahrq.gov>

5. Weiner, Jonathan P., DrPH. "Something 'Nice' Can Come Out of This." *Managed Care,* (January 2002).

6. Personal communication. E-mail exchange on PNHP's "Quote of the Day" (August 9, 2001). In Dr. Reinhardt's words: "The real explanation is that the American people prefer a health system whose costs rise in the high double digits. They fought for it at the job and in the political forum. Now they have it. Mazel tov!"

7. Callahan, David. *False Hopes. Why America's Quest for Perfect Health Is a Recipe for Failure.* Simon and Schuster. (1998).

8. *The Oregonian,* (December 20, 2001). Brandy's surgery, however, was to be covered by private funds raised with the help of a rich benefactor.

9. Leonhardt, David. "Health Care As Main Engine: Is That So Bad?" Money & Business Section. *The New York Times,* (November 11, 2001).

CHAPTER 12

1. Before a panel discussing House Concurrent Resolution 99, the "Health Care Access Resolution." (April 30, 2002).

2. Speaking before a panel discussion on House Concurrent Resolution 99, the "Health Care Access Resolution." (April 30, 2002).

3. Michels, R., et al. "Views of Managed Care." *New England Journal of Medicine* 340(12) (March 25,1999): 928.

4. Putnam, Robert. "A Better Society in a Time of War." Op-Ed. *The New York Times,* (October 19, 2001).

CHAPTER 13

1. As quoted in the *Cedar Rapids Gazette,* (April 19, 2002).

2. See: Goldfield, Norbert, MD. *National Health Reform American Style: Lessons from the Past. A Twentieth Century Journey.* American College of Physician Executives. (2000).

3. Ivins, Molly. "Health Care Rx: Phase Out the Failing For-Profit System." *Boulder Daily Camera,* (March 28, 2002).

CHAPTER 14

1. Miller, Joel E. "A Perfect Storm: the Confluence of Forces Affecting Health Care Coverage." National Coalition on Health Care. (November 2001).

2. Shuler, Marsha. "Breaux Favors Health Aid. Senator Backs Universal Coverage for All U.S. Citizens." *The Advocate Online*, (January 3, 2002).

3. See: <www.coveringtheuninsured.org>. The organizations include the U.S. Chamber of Commerce, the AFL-CIO, the Business Roundtable, the SEIU (Service Employees International Union), the American Medical Association, the American Nurses Association, the HIAA, Families USA, the American Hospital Association, the Federation of American Hospitals, the Catholic Health Association of the U.S., AARP, and the Robert Wood Johnson Foundation.

4. Belluck, Pam. "Small Vote for Universal Care Is Seen as Carrying a Lot of Weight." *The New York Times,* (November 16, 2001).

5. As an example, the coveringtheuninsured.org campaign is trying to educate the public about how the uninsured do poorly, die more frequently, and go bankrupt from medical bills. They also have publicized how 80 percent of the uninsured are in working families.

6. For a discussion of the possible role of civil disobedience in health care reform, see: Goldfield, Norbert, MD. *National Health Care Reform American Style: Lessons from the Past. A Twentieth Century Journey.* American College of Physician Executives. (2000).

CHAPTER 15

1. Meyer, Jack A.; Wicks, Elliott K. "Covering America. Real Remedies for the Uninsured." Economic and Social Research Institute. (June 2001).

2. Economic Policy Institute. *Paycheck Economics.* "Medicare at the Crossroads. Vouchers Take Us in the Wrong Direction." (March 2001).

3. See: <www.coveringtheuninsured.org>.

4. Collins, Karen Scott, et al. "Diverse Communities, Common Concerns: Assessing Health Care Quality for Minority Americans." See: <www.cmwf.org> .

5. Michels, R., et al. "Views of Managed Care." *New England Journal of Medicine* 340(12) (March 25, 1999): 928.

6. Himmelstein, David; Woolhandler, Steffie. *Bleeding the Patient.* Common Courage Press, Monroe, ME. (2001): p. 159.

7. Miller, Joel. "A Perfect Storm: the Confluence of Forces Affecting Health Care Coverage." National Coalition on Health Care. (November 2001).

CHAPTER 16

1. MSNBC's website carried an opinion piece from Art Caplan in September 2001 in which Art drew attention to the plight of the uninsured. He advocated for universal coverage, and doing it soon, through the use of government vouchers. This chapter responds to Art's assertion that "Single payer will not fly." My purpose is not so much to disagree with Art as to discuss the political, economic, and ethical relevance of universal coverage with a single-payer type approach. As explained in this chapter, approaches such as government vouchers are quick fixes, which would only make our already chaotic system more chaotic.

CHAPTER 17

1. "Study finds each pack of smokes costs nation $7 in care," *The Oregonian*, (April 12, 2002).

2. Reed, Marie C; Tu, Ha T. "Triple Jeopardy: Low Income, Chronically Ill, and Uninsured." Issue Brief No. 49. Center for Studying Health Care System Change. (February 2002).

3. Knowler, William C., et al. "Reduction in the Incidence of Type 2 Diabetes with Lifestyle Intervention or Metformin." *New England Journal of Medicine* 346(6) (February 7, 2002): 393-403.

4. Mokdad, Ali H., PhD., et al. "The Continuing Epidemics of Obesity and Diabetes in the United States." *JAMA* 286(10) (September 10, 2001): 1195-1200.

5. OECD (Organisation for Economic Co-operation and Development). "Health at a Glance." Paris. (2001). For people over 15 years old, the figures show that 25.1 percent of American females (and 19.9 percent of American males) have a BMI over 30. Both are much higher than the numbers for the other 23 countries.

6. Efforts to expel fast food from schools are happening around the country. Texas and California (among other places) are moving to ban junk foods from schools. On the national front, there is Congressional action with the Obesity Prevention and Treatment Act, introduced in May 2002. See: Egan, Timothy. "In a Bid to Improve Nutrition, Schools Expel Soda and Chips." *The New York Times*, (May 20, 2002).

7. For a more complete discussion of what has happened to food in America, see (1) Nestle, Marion, PhD, MPH. *Food Politics. How the Food Industry Influences Nutrition and Health.* University of California Press. (2002) and (2) Schlosser, Eric. *Fast Food Nation: The Dark Side of the All-American Meal.* Houghton Mifflin. (2001).

8. A comprehensive list of policy recommendations to reduce the prevalence of obesity (as well as ideas to promote physical activity) appears in: Nestle, Marion, PhD, MPH; Jacobson, Michael F., PhD. "Halting the Obesity Epidemic: A Public Health Approach." *Public Health Reports* 115 (January/February 2000). Also, the CDC's October 26, 2001, issue of MMWR, entitled "Increasing Physical Activity: A Report on Recommendations of the Task Force on Community Preventive Services," is devoted to an analysis of the options for promoting physical activity.

CHAPTER 18

1. An Institute of Medicine study released in March 2002 documented that minorities in America "receive lower quality health care than whites, even when their insurance and income are the same." From *The New York Times,* (March 21, 2002).

2. Ehrenreich, Barbara. *Nickel and Dimed. On (Not) Getting By in America.* Metropolitan Books. Henry Holt and Company, New York. (2001).

3. Ibid.

Selected Bibliography

Keeping Up to Date on Health Care Reform

The Kaiser Daily Health Policy Report
    <www.kaisernetwork.org/daily_reports/rep_hpolicy.cfm>
Kaiser Family Foundation website: <www.kff.org>
The Commonwealth Fund website: <www.cmwf.org>
Physicians for a National Health Program website: <www.pnhp.org>
Breaking news website: <www.everybodyinnobodyout.org>
American Medical News: <www.amednews.com>

Comprehensive Analysis and Data on the U.S. Health Care System

(These sources include a comprehensive overview of health care policy and cover the full range of topics that are listed separately below.)

Bodenheimer, Thomas S., MD; Grumbach, Kevin, MD.
    Understanding Health Policy. A Clinical Approach. Lange
    Medical Books. McGraw-Hill. Third Edition (2002).

Geyman, John P., MD. *Health Care in America. Can Our Ailing
    System Be Healed?* Butterworth/Heinemann. (2002).

Himmelstein, David, MD; Woolhandler, Steffie, MD, MPH; Hellander,
    Ida, MD. *Bleeding the Patient.* Common Courage Press, Monroe,
    ME. (2001).

Institute of Medicine website: <www.iom.edu/>

Kaiser Family Foundation. "Trends and Indicators in the Changing
    Health Care Marketplace 2002. Chartbook. (May 2002). See:
    <www.kff.org>

Kaiser Family Foundation website: <www.kff.org>

Mueller, Rudolph, MD. *As Sick as It Gets.* Olin Frederick, Inc.,
    Dunkirk, NY. (2001).

Health Care Policy

Angell, Marcia, MD. "Patients' Rights Bills and Other Futile
    Gestures." *New England Journal of Medicine* 342(22) (June 1,
    2000): 1663-1664.

Garrett, Laurie. *Betrayal of Trust: The Collapse of Global Public
    Health.* Hyperion, New York. (2000).

Kleinke, J.D. *Oxymorons: The Myth of the U.S. Health Care System.* Jossey-Bass. (2001).

McCanne, Don, MD. "Why Incremental Reforms Will Not Solve the Health Care Crisis." The Journal of the American Board of Family Practice 16 (2003): 257-261. <www.jabfp.org/cgi/content/full/16/3/257>

McDonough, John E., DrPH. *Healthcare Policy. The Basics.* The Access Project. (1999).

Miller, Joel E. "A Perfect Storm: The Confluence of Forces Affecting Health Care Coverage." National Coalition on Health Care. (November 2001).

Oberlander, Jonathan B.; Marmor, Theodore R. "The Path to Universal Health Care." (2000).

O'Connor, Kathleen, MA. *The Buck Stops Nowhere. Why America's Healthcare is All Dollars and No Sense.* Hara Publishing Group, Seattle. (April 2001).

The Uninsured

American College of Physicians – American Society of Internal Medicine. "No Health Insurance? It's Enough to Make You Sick—Scientific Research Linking the Lack of Health Coverage to Poor Health."(2000). Available at: <www.acponline.org/uninsured/>

Ayanian, John Z., MD, MPP, et al. "Unmet Health Needs of Uninsured Adults in the United States." *JAMA* 284(16) (October 25, 2000): 2061-2069.

Bell, Howard. "Life Without Insurance: True Stories of Unnecessary Sickness, Death and Humiliation." *The New Physician* (AMSA). (September 2000).

Bodenheimer, Thomas, MD, MPH. "Underinsurance in America." *New England Journal of Medicine* 327(4). (July 23, 1992): 274-278.

Commonwealth Fund website: <www.cmwf.org>

Ferrer, Robert L., MD, MPH. "A Piece of My Mind. Within the System of No-System." *JAMA* 286(20) (November 28, 2001): 2513-2514.

Franks, Peter, MD; Clancy, Carolyn, M., MD; Gold, Marthe R., MPH. "Health Insurance and Mortality." *JAMA* 270(6) (August 11, 1993): 737-741.

Geyman, J.P. *Falling Through the Safety Net: Americans Confront the Perils of Health Insurance.* Monroe, Me.: Common Courage Press, 2004

Grumbach, Kevin, MD. "Insuring the Uninsured. Time to End the Aura of Invisibility." *JAMA* 284(16) (October 25, 2000): 2114-2116.

Institute of Medicine. *Care Without Coverage: Too Little, Too Late.* National Academy Press, Washington, D.C. (May 2002).

Kaiser Commission on Medicaid and the Uninsured. "Sicker and Poorer: The Consequences of Being Uninsured." (May 2002). <www.kff.org>

Reed, Marie C.; Tu, Ha T. "Triple Jeopardy: Low Income, Chronically Ill, and Uninsured in America." Issue Brief No. 49. Center for Studying Health System Change. (February 2002). <www.hschange.org>

Rowland, Diane, ScD. The Kaiser Commission on Medicaid and the Uninsured. "The New Challenge of the Uninsured: Coverage in the Current Economy." Testimony for the "Uninsured and Affordable Health Care Coverage" Subcommittee on Health. Committee on Energy and Commerce. U.S. House of Representatives. (February 28, 2002). <www.kff.org>

"Second-Class Medicine." *Consumer Reports*, (September 2000): 42-50.

History of Health Care Reform in America

Davis, Karen. "Universal Coverage in the United States: Lessons From Experience of the 20th Century." *Journal of Urban Health: Bulletin of the New York Academy of Medicine* 78 (March 2001): 46-58.

Goldfield, Norbert, MD. *National Health Care Reform American Style: Lessons from the Past. A Twentieth Century Journey.* American College of Physician Executives. (2000).

Oberlander, J. *The Political Life of Medicare.* Chicago: University of Chicago Press, 2003

Sigerist, H.E. Medical Care for all the People. *Canadian Journal of Public Health*, 35(7), 258, 1944.

Starr, P. *The Social Transformation of American Medicine.* New York, Basic Books, 1982, pp.252-3.

Proposals for Health Care Reform

American Academy of Family Physicians. "Assuring Health Care Coverage for All." (October 2001). See: <www.aafp.org/unicov/hccfa.pdf>

American College of Physicians – American Society of Internal Medicine. "Achieving Affordable Health Insurance for All Within Seven Years." (April 9, 2002). See: <www.acponline.org/hpp/afford—7years.pdf>

Angell, Marcia, MD. "Dispelling the Myths About Single-Payer Health Care." Newsletter of the Universal Health Care Education Fund. (November 2001).

Bodenheimer, T. The Movement for Universal Health Insurance: Finding Common Ground. *American Journal of Public Health*, 93, 112, 2003.

California Health Care Options Project; preliminary-full drafts of each proposal are available at http://www.healthcareoptions.ca.gov/doclib.asp, 2002.

Caplan, Art, PhD. "New World Calls for New Health Care. Government Should Provide Safety Net for All Americans." (September 28, 2001). <www.msnbc.com/news/635352>

Commonwealth Fund website: <www.cmwf.org>

Davis, Karen, PhD; Schoen, Cathy, MS; Schoenbaum, Stephen C., MD, MPH. "A 2020 Vision for American Health Care." *Archives of Internal Medicine* 160(22) (December 11/25, 2000).

Economic Policy Institute. *Paycheck Economics.* "Medicare at the Crossroads. Vouchers Take Us in the Wrong Direction." (March 2001).

Evans, R.G., Going for the Gold: The redistributive agenda behind market-based health care reform. *Journal of Health Politics, Policy and Law* 22(2),427, 1997.

Geyman, J.P. Family Practice in a Failing Health Care System: New Opportunities to Advocate for System Reform, *Journal of American Board of Family Practice*, 2002;15(5):407-16.

Geyman, J.P. Myths as Barriers to Health Care Reform in the U.S. *International Journal of Health Services*, 2003,33(2);315-29.

Glied, Sherry A. "Challenges and Options for Increasing the Number of Americans With Health Insurance." The Commonwealth Fund. (January 2001).

Himmelstein, David U., MD; Woolhandler, Steffie, MD, MPH, et al. "A National Health Program for the United States. A Physicians' Proposal." *New England Journal of Medicine* 320 (January 12, 1989): 102-108.

Himmelstein, David U., MD; Woolhandler, Steffie, MD, MPH. "National Health Insurance. Liberal Benefits, Conservative Spending." *Archives of Internal Medicine* 162 (May 13, 2002): 973-975.

Institute of Medicine. "Insuring America's Health: Principles and Recommendations."(January 14, 2004).<www.iom.edu/report:asp?id=17632>

Kahn, Charles N., III; Pollack, Ronald F. "Building a Consensus for Expanding Health Coverage." *Health Affairs* 20 (1) (January/February 2001): 40-48.

Light, Donald W. "Health Care for All: A Conservative Case." *Commonweal*, (February 22, 2002).

Meyer, Jack A.; Wicks, Elliot K. *Covering America. Real Remedies for the Uninsured.* Economic and Social Research Institute. (June 2001).

Physicians for a National Health Program website: <www.pnhp.org>

"Proposal of the Physicians' Working Group for Single-Payer National Health Insurance." JAMA 290 (6) (August 13, 2003): 798-805. www.physiciansproposal.org/proposal/Physicians%20ProposalJA MA.pdf

The Future of Health Insurance in the U.S.

Fuchs, Victor R., PhD. "What's Ahead for Health Insurance in the United States?" *New England Journal of Medicine* 346(23) (June 6, 2002): 1822-1824.

"The Unraveling of Health Insurance." *Consumer Reports*, (July 2002): 48-53.

Public Health

Garrett, Laurie. *Betrayal of Trust: The Collapse of Global Public Health.* Hyperion, New York. (2000).

Prevention (Obesity and Physical Activity)

MMWR (Morbidity and Mortality Weekly Report). "Increasing Physical Activity: A Report on Recommendations of the Task Force on Community Preventive Services." Vol. 50. No. RR18; 1. (October 26, 2001).

Mokdad, Ali H., PhD, et al. "The Continuing Epidemics of Obesity and Diabetes in the United States." *JAMA* 286(10) (September 12, 2001): 1195-1200.

Mokdad, Ali H., PhD, et al. "The Spread of the Obesity Epidemic in the United States, 1991-1998." *JAMA* 282(16) (October 27, 1999): 1519-1522.

Nelson, David E., et al. "State Trends in Health Risk Factors and Receipt of Clinical Preventive Services Among U.S. Adults During the 1990's." *JAMA* 287(20) (May 22/29, 2002): 2659-2667.

Nestle, Marion, PhD, MPH. *Food Politics. How the Food Industry Influences Nutrition and Health.* University of California Press. (2002).

Nestle, Marion, PhD, MPH; Jacobson, Michael F., PhD. "Halting the Obesity Epidemic: A Public Health Policy Approach." *Public Health Reports* 115. (January/February 2000): 15-24.

Schlosser, Eric. *Fast Food Nation: The Dark Side of the All-American Meal.* Houghton Mifflin, Boston. (2001).

Strauss, Richard S., MD; Pollack, Harold A, PhD. "Epidemic Increase in Childhood Overweight, 1986-1998." *JAMA* 286(22) (December 12, 2001): 2845-2848.

Ethics in Health Care

Callahan, Daniel. *False Hopes*. Simon & Schuster. (1998).

Light, D.W. The Practice and Ethics of Risk-Related Health Insurance. JAMA 267,2503, 1992.

Pellegrino, E.D. The Commodification of Medical and Health Care: The Moral Consequences of a Paradigm Shift from a Professional to a Market Ethic. *Journal of Medical Philosophy*, 1999;24:243-66.

Reinhardt, Uwe E., PhD. "Wanted: A Clearly Articulated Social Ethic for American Health Care." *JAMA* 278(17) (November 5, 1997): 1446-1447.

Sider, Ronald J. Chapter 6: "Does Justice Include Health Care for the Poor?" *Just Generosity. A New Vision for Overcoming Poverty in America*. Baker Books, Grand Rapids, Mich. (1999).

Fraud

Sparrow, Malcolm K. *License to Steal. How Fraud Bleeds America's Health Care System*. Westview Press. (2000).

Health Care in Other Countries

Anderson, Gerard; Hussey, Peter Sotir. "Comparing Health System Performance In OECD Countries." *Health Affairs* (May/June 2001).

Armstrong, Pat; Armstrong, Hugh; with Fegan, Claudia, MD. *Universal Health Care. What the United States Can Learn From the Canadian Experience*. The New Press, New York. (1998).

Commission on the Future of Health Care in Canada <www.hc-sc.gc.ca/english/care/romanow/index1.html>

Organization for Economic Cooperation and Development (OECD), Health Data 2001. See: <www.oecd.org>

Rice, Thomas, et al. "Special Section: Reconsidering the Role of Competition in Health Care Markets." *Journal of Health Politics, Policy, and Law* 25 (5) (October 2000): 863-978.

Saltman, Richard B.; Figueras, Josep. "Analyzing the Evidence on European Health Care Reforms." *Health Affairs* 17(2) (March/April 1998): 85-108.

Starfield, Barbara, MD, MPH. "Is US Health Really the Best in the World?" *JAMA* 284(4) (July 26, 2000): 483-485.

World Health Organization. *The World Health Report 2000. Health Systems: Improving Performance*. Geneva. (2000).

Medicare and Medicaid

Boccuti,C. & Moon,M. Comparing Medicare and Private Insurers: Growth Rates in Spending over Three Decades. *Health Affairs(Millwood)*, 22(2),230, 2003.

Bodenheimer,T. The Dismal Failures of Medicare Privatization. Senior Action Network, San Francisco,1, June 2003.

Dao, James. "On the Streets of Baltimore, the Word on Medicare Is 'Expand,' Not 'Overhaul'." *The New York Times*, (September 8, 2000).

Economic Policy Institute. *Paycheck Economics.* "Medicare at the Crossroads. Vouchers Take Us in the Wrong Direction." (March 2001).

Kaiser Family Foundation website: <www.kff.org>

Public Citizen Report. Medicare Privatization: The Case Against Relying on the HMOs and Private Insurers to Offer Prescription Drug Coverage, 2002. Available on the Web at www.citizen.org/congress/reform/rx_benefits/drug_benefit/articles.cfm?ID-8298. Accessed October 2, 2003.

Health Care Costs, Co-Payments

Blumenthal, David, MD, MPP. "Controlling Health Care Expenditures." *New England Journal of Medicine* 344(10) (March 8, 2001): 766-769.

Grumbach, K. & Bodenheimer, T. Reins or Fences: A Physicians's View of Cost Containment. *Health Affairs(Millwood)* 1990;9:120-6.

Kolata, Gina. "Medical Fees Are Often More For Uninsured." *The New York Times,* (April 2, 2001).

Rasell, M. Edith, MD. "Cost Sharing in Health Insurance—a Reexamination." *New England Journal of Medicine* 332(17) (April 27, 1995).

Tamblyn, R.; Laprise, R.; Hanley, JA, et al. "Adverse Effects Associated with Prescription Drug Cost-Sharing Among Poor and Elderly Persons." *JAMA* 285(2001): 421-429.

Wielawski, Irene. "Gouging the Medically Uninsured: A Tale of Two Bills." *Health Affairs* 19(5) (September/October 2000): 180-185.

Woolhandler, S. & Himmelstein, D.U. Paying for National Health Insurance—and not Getting it. *Health Affairs(Millwood)* 21(4) 88, 2002a.

Woolhandler, S., MD,MPH;Campbell, T.,MHA; Himmelstein, D.U., MD. "Costs of Health Care Administration in the United States and Canada." *New England Journal of Medicine* 349(August 21, 2003): 768-775.

Business and Health Care

Anthony, Joseph. "The Answer for Small Business: Guaranteed Health Care."(December 2001).
<Microsoft.bcentral.com/articles/Anthony/166>

Geyman, J.P. The Corporate Transformation of Medicine and its Impact on Costs and Access to Care. *Journal of American Board of Family Practice*, 2003; 16,443-454.

Gleckman, Howard. "The Nasty Side Effects of Medical Savings Accounts." *Business Week*, (October 25, 1999): 42.

Kuttner, Robert. "A Dirty Little Secret: Managed Care is Bad for Business." *Business Week*, (December 21, 1998).

Kuttner, Robert. "The American Health Care System—Employer-Sponsored Health Coverage." *New England Journal of Medicine* 340(3) (January 21, 1999): 248-252.

Kuttner, R. *Everything for Sale: The Virtues and Limits of Markets*. Chicago: University of Chicago Press, 1999.

Kuttner, R. Must Good HMOs Go Bad? First of Two Parts: the Commercialism of Prepaid Group Health Care. *New England Journal of Medicine*, 1998;338:1558-63.

Woolhandler, S. & Himmelstein, D.U. When Money is the Mission—The High Costs of Investor-owned Care. *New England Journal of Medicine*, 1999;341:444-6.

The Pharmaceutical Industry

Angell, Marcia, MD. "The Pharmaceutical Industry—to Whom Is It Accountable?" *New England Journal of Medicine* 342(25) (June 22, 2000): 1902-1904.

Angell, M. & Relman, A.S. Prescription for Profit. www.washington-post.com. June 21, 2001.

Baker, D. Patent Medicine. *The American Prospect*. January 29, 2001, pp 34-5.

Bodenheimer, Thomas S., MD. "Affordable Prescriptions for the Elderly." *JAMA* 286(14) (October 10, 2001): 1762-1763.

Little, Shannon. "Public Citizen Report Debunks R&D Myths. Rx Drug Industry Exaggerates Costs, Blocks Efforts to Lower Drug Prices." *Public Citizen News*, (September/October 2001): 4.

Mueller, Rudolph, MD. *As Sick as It Gets*. Chapter 4. Olin Frederick, Inc., Dunkirk, NY. (2001). Website: <www.nofreelunch.org>

Appendix

Frequently Asked Questions (FAQs)
About "One Risk Pool"

Q. What defines "one risk pool"?

A risk pool is an insurance term used to describe a group of people who are all insured in the same group and, thus, share coverage and risk. The risk pool lumps them all together so no one person can be "wiped out" financially in case of a health catastrophe. Health care providers also are assured of payment. If there were "one risk pool" that included all 280 million people in America in the same group, the risk would be maximally shared. This would essentially constitute a form of national health insurance with universal coverage.

Q. Is "one risk pool" the same as "single payer"?

Not exactly, though it could be. "One risk pool" refers to the group of people—in this case all Americans—enrolled in the plan. "Single payer" refers to a payment mechanism, where one entity, usually government, has the responsibility for paying the bills. It would be possible, though administratively more complex, to have multiple payers for a single risk pool.

Q. How is "one risk pool" similar to Medicare?

Medicare is a single risk pool for all Americans 65 years old and older (and a few other categories). For those 65 and over, the eligibility is universal and the enrollment automatic. In contrast, the proposed single risk pool includes everyone (all ages) in America. And the proposed single risk pool would have a more comprehensive range of benefits than the current Medicare.

Q. How would a "one risk pool" system be financed?

The overall financing would be similar to Medicare. But unlike traditional insurance (and to some extent Medicare) with its premiums, deductibles, and co-pays, the funding would come almost exclusively through progressive taxation, with everyone paying into a trust fund according to his/her ability to pay. It is not free.

Q. What is the role of government in the "one risk pool" approach?

Government would collect the taxes, assure the trust fund is solvent, oversee the system administratively, contract out for payments to providers, assure that guidelines are set for the benefit plan, and provide accountability to the American people for the functioning of the system. The delivery system would remain predominantly private, as is today.

Q. What would happen to the insurance companies under "one risk pool"?

The insurance companies would perform contracted administrative functions for the plan. They would be able to sell insurance for benefits not covered under the plan.

Q. What kind of benefit package would a system with "one risk pool" have?

It would be a comprehensive package, encompassing all "necessary" care, including inpatient and ambulatory care, emergency care, mental health, diagnostic testing, basic dental health, long-term care, eye care, and medical equipment. There would be no deductibles, and no co-pays except for services deemed to be "marginal."

Q. Who would decide what the benefits would be with "one risk pool"?

The benefits package would be developed primarily through a consensus of the American people with the collaboration of "boards of health," both national and regional (or state). Priorities, guidelines, and global budgets will need to be set.

Q. How could such a generous benefit package be affordable with "one risk pool"?

"One risk pool" makes such a rich package affordable because of the vastly decreased administrative costs and the elimination of middlemen. These savings should amount to over $200 billion (2002 estimate)—more than enough to provide the resources needed to cover every person in America. Global budgeting helps to assure a cap on the spending.

Q. Wouldn't "choice" be decreased with "one risk pool"?

The opposite is true. There would in fact be more choice, as a person could go to any provider of his/her choice—including an HMO.

Q. Would someone be able to "opt out" of the pool and get "extra" care?

Hopefully the "one risk pool" approach will be comprehensive enough and of high enough quality that there would be no need or desire to "opt out." However, anyone could buy supplemental insurance or pay out of pocket for services that are not covered. Beyond those limited circumstances, it will be up to the American people to decide whether to include "a safety valve" in the design of the plan—at the risk of creating a multi-tiered system.

Q. Would the "pool" include illegal immigrants?

A whole topic in itself. The short answer is "yes." These people do some of the most dangerous and difficult jobs in our society.

They contribute more to our economy than they take out. And corporations that hire them often fail to provide them with health insurance, thus shifting the cost of their health care to taxpayers in general. The humanitarian answer is also "yes."

Q. Is it fair that someone who doesn't work and contribute to the trust fund gets a "free ride"?

The question reflects an "anti-welfare" sentiment expressed by many Americans. It brings into question the very existence of our current Medicaid program and ignores the fact that 80 percent of Americans who are uninsured are part of a working family. It also fails to recognize that everyone in America pays some taxes, be it sales tax, gasoline tax, or rent (which includes the landlord's real estate tax). And it overlooks the sad truth that many people are unable to work because of disabilities for which they're unable to get medical care. An example of "blaming the victim."

Q. What would we do with all the administrative people who would lose their jobs if we had a single risk pool? Wouldn't there be an economic disaster?

These people could be retrained to do useful work in the health care system, such as outreach, health education, and the provision of transportation. They would help meet the unmet needs. One example: nurses who now spend their time doing administrative work could once again do nursing.

Q. Isn't "one risk pool" the same as socialized medicine?

No. "One risk pool" is an insurance arrangement that allows huge administrative savings and enrollment equity—with everyone included and no one left out. The physicians and hospitals would be largely independent and not employed or owned by the government, as they are in the U.K., which has a system based primarily on socialized medicine.

Glossary of Terms

AAFP: The American Academy of Family Physicians

ACP-ASIM: American College of Physicians/American Society of Internal Medicine. The specialists in internal medicine.

AMA: The American Medical Association

AMSA: American Medical Student Association

ANA: American Nurses Association

AHRQ: Agency for Health Care Research and Quality

BBA: The Balanced Budget Amendment (1997)

CDC: The Centers for Disease Control and Prevention

CHCs: Community Health Centers, a federally-funded national program to expand access to care for poor and rural populations. They offer a sliding-fee scale for payment based on income, and are often referred to as "safety-net" clinics.

CHIP: see SCHIP

CMS: Center for Medicare and Medicaid Services, formerly HCFA, or the Health Care Financing Administration.

DRG: Diagnosis Related Groups, whereby a hospital is paid a set fee for a particular diagnosis.

ER: Emergency Room

GAO: General Accounting Office

GDP: Gross Domestic Product

HCFA: Health Care Financing Administration, since 2001 renamed CMS, or Center for Medicare and Medicaid Services

HHS: Health and Human Services

HIAA: Health Insurance Association of America

HMO: Health Maintenance Organization

273

HRSA: The Health Resources Service Administration. A federal agency that is part of Health and Human Services.

JAMA: Journal of the American Medical Association

Medicaid: The federal/state health insurance program, initiated in 1965, that covers poor Americans, most nursing home costs, and a few other groups. Costs are shared between the federal and state governments. Eligibility varies from state to state.

Medicare: The federal health insurance program, also initiated in 1965, that covers people 65 and older, some disabled people, and people receiving renal dialysis.

MRI scan: Magnetic Resonance Imagery, a relative of X-rays. It can be used to diagnose soft-tissue problems as well as abnormalities of bones.

MSA: Medical Savings Account

NACHC: National Association of Community Health Centers

NHI: National Health Insurance

OECD: Organisation for Economic Co-operation and Development

PET scan: Positron Emission Tomography, a new and more expensive version of the MRI

PHS: Public Health Service

PNHP: Physicians for a National Health Program, a national organization, started in 1987, of over 9000 members advocating for single-payer national health insurance.

PPO: Physician Provider Organization

R&D: Research and Development

SCHIP or CHIP: The (State) Children's Health Insurance Program, initiated in 1997, that expands coverage to near low-income children whose families earn too much for them to qualify for Medicaid. Some states have expanded CHIP to include the parents.

UHCAN: Universal Health Coverage for America Network

USPSTF: U.S. Preventive Services Task Force

WHO: The World Health Organization

Index

About the Author

Bob LeBow, MD, MPH, was the Medical Director of a community health center in Idaho for over 25 years. A graduate of Harvard College and the Johns Hopkins School of Medicine, Dr. LeBow was board certified in two specialties: family practice and preventive medicine. He had extensive experience working on the development of health systems and preventive programs in over 20 developing countries, including a two-year stint as a Peace Corps physician in Bolivia.

Dr. LeBow, however, devoted most of his career to addressing the problems of health care in the United States. A self-described "health care activist," in 1998 and 1999 he was president of Physicians for a National Health Program.

After having been paralyzed in a cycling accident, he died in late 2003.